ADVANCED PRAISE

"At this critical time, women are in dire need of true, loving leadership to break-free from fear and step into their authentic power. Kate Dow offers that openhearted, knowing leadership. She speaks with clarity and wisdom to the places we struggle, then navigates us through new life affirming pathways with skill and care. Every woman who wants to live with peace, inner strength, personal power and deeper connection with themselves and others, needs to read this book and make it part of their life."

- GINI GENTRY, a Nagual woman, author
of *Dreaming Down Heaven*

"This book is full of practical tools and most of all loving support and direction as you learn to return to a life of calm and joy. It feels like Kate is right there with you, holding your heart and your hand."

- KIRN KHALSA, co-author of *Numerology for Self-Mastery*, owner of Purest Potential

"In one short sentence, Dr. Dow summarizes the key to banishing anxiety: "Self-care starves anxiety." But how many women really know what self-care means? The Fear-Less Path is a three-pronged approach for helping talented female entrepreneurs break free of anxiety so they can get their messages out into the world. Utilizing the practices detailed here for mind, body, and spirit, women can reclaim their feminine power, voice and creativity. Here they can truly shine, free from anxiety."

- JEANNE ANDRUS, The Menopause Guru,
Author *of I Just Want to Be ME Again! A
Guide to Thriving Through Menopause*

"We all have experienced anxiety along with stress in our lives. We tend to override it and keep going. Now here's a concept: Use the energy of anxiety to meet your goals. The author uses the archetypes of the Queen, the Heroine and the Goddess self to specifically support women in this endeavor. She offers dynamic practices that empower us to evolve and restore control of our lives and purpose. This is particularly useful for those of us working to bring change about politically. We need all the tools we can get!"

- MARILYN ROSENBROCK NYBORG,
Co-founder of Indivisible Women of Nevada
County, soon to be published author: *A Women's Guide to Sacred Activism*

"From her deep roots in spiritual wisdom traditions, decades in the field of Counseling Psychology, as well her own lived experience, Dr. Kate Dow offers a book that goes straight to the core and is full of practical tools for women living with anxiety. As she guides the reader, with unwavering compassion and clarity, to connect with resources we all have within us, reading this book becomes a profoundly empowering journey."

-CHAMELI ARDAGH, Author of
Embodying the Feminine, Founder of
AwakeningWomen.com

FEAR-LESS

FEAR-LESS

The Art of Using Your Anxiety
to Your Advantage

Dr. KATE DOW

NEW YORK

LONDON • NASHVILLE • MELBOURNE • VANCOUVER

Fear-Less

The Art of Using Your Anxiety to Your Advantage

Published in New York, New York, by Morgan James Publishing in partnership with Difference Press. Morgan James is a trademark of Morgan James, LLC.
www.MorganJamesPublishing.com

The Morgan James Speakers Group can bring authors to your live event. For more information or to book an event visit The Morgan James Speakers Group at www.TheMorganJamesSpeakersGroup.com.

ISBN 9781642790245 paperback
ISBN 9781642790252 eBook
Library of Congress Control Number: 2018937252

Cover Design by:
Megan Dillon
megan@creativeninjadesigns.com

Interior Design by:
Chris Treccani
www.3dogcreative.net

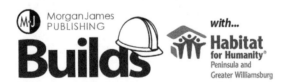

In an effort to support local communities, raise awareness and funds, Morgan James Publishing donates a percentage of all book sales for the life of each book to Habitat for Humanity Peninsula and Greater Williamsburg.

Get involved today! Visit
www.MorganJamesBuilds.com

To all women, with my love, honor, and admiration.
"May we step into our hearts and our courage
with fierce devotion,
May we own our voices and our gifts with divine respect,
May we heal ourselves and support one another
with gentle compassion,
May we find our inner peace and know our deepest True Selves,
Then, surely, we can save humanity and this precious place,
Mother Earth, we call Home."

– Dr. Kate Dow

TABLE OF CONTENTS

PART ONE

"Life presents us with repeated opportunities to face what we fear, what we need to become conscious of, or what we need to master."

– Jean Shiboda Bolen

THE CHALLENGES OF ANXIETY

"Too many of us are not living our dreams
because we are living our fears."
– Les Brown

Welcome amazing women, I am so glad you are here. We have all traveled far in our lives to get here. It's time for healing now. I truly know how devastating and challenging anxiety can be. I wrote this book especially for us, women with anxiety, who have struggled to find the way to get rid of it once and for all. We all deserve to live free of fear and anxiety running our lives. In the stress of having anxiety, we can get too focused on our problems, fears, and worries, and lose sight of how life could be different. If you have tried methods that have helped your anxiety for a while but didn't last, you are in the right place.

There are millions of women with anxiety(1). Living in this culture that is fast-paced, high stress, and focused on perfection, power, and control is enough to bring most of us anxiety. Add on feminine oppression and/or childhood trauma, and that pretty much covers the rest of us. Women are feeling fearful and isolated, believing it's only happening to themselves. This is tragic and not OK. We are in this together, and need to know we matter and can get help. In this day and age, why should people have to suffer when there are so many non-medical methods that actually can help? We just haven't heard about them, and it's hard to know what is good information. This is why I wrote this book.

Just so you know, it's not our fault we are suffering. We all do the best we can with what we know. Making a change once we have the correct information about our anxiety then becomes our choice. We each get to decide whether we are sick enough of anxiety to make the necessary changes. A lot of fears can show up just by thinking about change, can't they? That's completely normal. We may start to wonder, "Is this worth it, trying to solve my anxiety again?" We could go back to believing that this is just the crappy way life is and it will never be any different. In other words, just keep suffering. That is a choice, even if it is a horrible one.

It is easy to stay in the familiar places we're stuck in, even if we know they are bad for us. We can't help it. We all have these lower, reptilian parts of our brains that prefer to just keep life the same, even if we're miserable. They were quite helpful back in the stone ages, when we needed to stay safe finding food and not get eaten by tigers. They know how we can stay "safe" as a baseline. The problem is that being "safe" does not mean happy or thriving. This is like life with anxiety: It's not very comfortable at all and actually very painful. However, the lower brain is satisfied with its target goal of just keeping you alive. It says anxiety is no big deal, as long as you are alive. Meanwhile, you feel exhausted, tense, irritable, lonely, sick of it, stressed, worried constantly, sleep-deprived, unhappy….

Sometimes we may try a new strategy for dealing with our anxiety and get good results, but our lower brain will eventually shut it down. This is a relative of the lower brain we call the ego mind: what I nickname "Our little personality's dictator." The ego wants to stay in charge, and the only way it can do that is if it stays more powerful than your conscious mind. The ego doesn't like us risking our perceived safety and comfort for freedom, empowerment, and a good life. It will align with our lower brain and stop us from changing. The ego is very skilled at coming up with all the reasons that a new idea is not worth the time, energy, or money to try to stop the pain of anxiety. It will say that it's pointless, that everything is just fine the way it is. And so, you return to life with anxiety running you, keeping you tense, agitated, unsure of yourself, worried, and self-conscious. It's brutal, isn't it? You don't even want others to know how hard it is for you to just get through the day, because you feel ashamed. Because you think you are the only one with this problem. Which of course is completely untrue.

Let's take a look at the real cost of staying in the unhelpful "safe" zone controlled by your little dictator and lower brain. How self-critical and hard on yourself are you because you haven't figured this anxiety thing out? How has the stress of anxiety impacted your health? We know stress correlates with increased inflammation, which makes us more vulnerable to getting illnesses(2). Does your anxiety start waking you up at night to tell you all the things you're not doing right and should be doing better? Is it getting harder to get through the day or week? Does your anxiety make it nearly impossible for you to drive? Is it getting tougher to do what you need to do at work? If you got a dream job offer right now, doing exactly what you love, would your ego and anxiety sabotage you and say, "You don't deserve that," or "You aren't good enough"? You just want to live your life and feel at peace, but fear and anxiety do the opposite, making you feel stressed out, worried, and not like yourself. And if you want to get out there and help people, as a coach or leader, but your anxiety is getting in the way of that happening, this is absolutely not acceptable anymore.

Here is my vision of your life without anxiety constantly messing with you. What if I said you could feel more peaceful, calm, and like yourself again? You would know how to handle your anxiety when it shows up so it couldn't sabotage you anymore. You would feel less on edge with whatever life threw at you and you would know what do when things did get overwhelming. Your sleep would be better and more regular. Worry would no longer suck all of your energy out of you. You would be able to drive with more ease and be social with friends. You would have the confidence, inner peace and self-esteem to follow your passion and get your message out there where it belongs You would have your life back and much more.

This sounds pretty good, right? As you read that description, did you notice your ego saying something like, "I don't know about this. How do we know it will work?" This means it doesn't *want* it to work. You see how sneaky the ego is? This book will show you how to rewire your brain so that the lower brain and ego no longer run the show. You get to create new neural pathways that can support the changes you want to make.

Let's cut to the chase. There are two types of fear in the world: helpful and unhelpful. The kind that keeps us from walking off the curb in front of a car is helpful. The kind that keeps us from living our life, telling us all the reasons we can't do it, is the unhelpful kind. This is the crossroads, where you have an important choice. You need to remember that you are in charge of your life. This is your life and no one else's. Be the queen of yourself for a moment.

To be your Queen Self, you must call an audience with only the parts of you that are intrigued and excited about this chance to stop anxiety from running your life. These are the parts of you that are already motivated and have energy to make this happen. These parts are inspired, despite the chatter of the lower brain and ego. They want to scream, "YES! We can do this!"

It's time to escape the anxiety lockdown you've been living in. This book is the key. Stay focused. Notice how the powerful parts of you are ready and want you to have the life that you've been wanting. Have them up front and speaking up the loudest in the audience of your mind. Mute the ego. Focus only on the drive and excitement of these powerful parts. They are going to rescue you from the prison of your lower brain. This is possible, if you are ready to put yourself at the top of the to-do list for a time. This book will show you the way.

Can you see it? Take a moment and picture this, because this is super important. Visualize yourself and your life a year from now, after you've learned how to deal with your anxiety. Who will you be without the weight and ruin of your anxiety running you? How will your life look and feel? How will you stand in your body? How will you be different when you wake up in the morning? How will you show up in the world differently? Visualize it now. This visualization exercise is powerful because we know the brain does not discern between "real" and "imagined." Our body and mind respond to guided imagery and imagination as if it was actually happening, leading to psychological and physiological changes(3). So, let's use this to our advantage. Tell yourself this is already happening now.

Accept this as your vision of what is possible. Breathe it into your lungs. Gently open your heart and accept that this is your future. That future is on the other side of the door of your life. It is time to walk through this door. The excited part of you that picked up this book is your life muse, and it's encouraging you to stop sitting on the sidelines of life and jump in as if you had nothing to lose. Be brave. I am with you.

Let's go. I want you to benefit and learn from my lifelong searches for how to overcome anxiety. Come, your anxiety-free life is waiting.

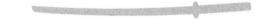

"The surest way to escape anxiety and defeat despair is action.
Do, don't dwell."
– Michael Josephson

CHAPTER 1

———

Your Uninvited Guest

"Our anxiety does not empty tomorrow of its sorrows,
but only empties today of its strengths."
– **Charles Spurgeon**

Let's get real about what living with anxiety is like. It doesn't seem to matter *when* anxiety enters your life, because once it does, it feels like it's been there forever, hiding out and springing up on you when you least expect it. You come to accept its presence, like a stayed-way-past-their-welcome guest in your home, that you think you just have to put up with. You think you must be a good host. You try to nicely ask it when it will be leaving. It doesn't work. You start to get a little snippy with it. What can you do? You feel trapped. You have somehow allowed this unseemly guest into your house and you cannot get rid of it. Who invited it anyway? Doesn't it know that this is your house?

You feel powerless over its presence in your life. It seems to be calling the shots more and more every time you look around. Now it's showing up in other areas of your life. It starts inviting itself to come with you to lunch with your friends, making you feel uncomfortable, tense, and worried you will say the wrong thing. Or it might tell you, "If someone asks you to help them, you'd better say 'yes' because you don't want to disappoint anybody." Even though you're tired, you agree to help a friend who needs help cleaning out her garage! You can hear anxiety, sounding just like your mother, saying, "Put others first, dear. Don't be selfish!" It keeps happening. You think, "No, I can't," but "Yes, sure, no problem" keeps coming out of your mouth. You feel stressed and out of control.

Now this uninvited guest is making you worry about the future. It's making things up to worry about and get insecure over. You aren't sure about any of it. Now it's creating distance between you and your friends and family. It's lonely. You feel all alone with this uninvited guest. Now it's showing up at your work. It begins questioning your ability to do the work that you've been doing for years. What's up with that? Next thing you know, you're asking yourself, "Am I really as good at this as I thought, or am I fooling myself?" The uninvited guest keeps expanding its territory of influence, which is devastating when you really want to help others and you know can, if you can get past this.

When chaos blows into your life, this guest chimes in with its critique of you, and begins talking about all of the worst-case scenarios. It is very disturbing. You are getting overwhelmed now. You feel so exhausted it's becoming worrisome. You notice you are being more critical and short-fused with your coworkers and family, and telling them things like "Just get it done."

But it doesn't go well. In fact, the more you push yourself and others, the more anxious you get. It seems that no matter how hard you try to pull up those bootstraps, it is just not working. You have no time for yourself. You feel lonely and estranged from people. Now your sleep is getting interrupted. The guest is showing up in your room at night, talking about the decisions you should rethink and do better. You start feeling bad about yourself. You never get a break. You feel awful in your body. You start worrying, "What is wrong with me?"

Nothing is wrong with you. You just need to learn how to send that uninvited guest packing. This book is the ticket. Then you can have yourself, your house, your mind, and your life back again. This approach gives you the steps to actually make this happen. It gives you the tools and experiences that help you sustain change in a way you never thought possible. It is quite possible, I promise.

"Change happens not by trying to make yourself change
but by becoming conscious of what's not working."
– Shakti Gawain

CHAPTER 2

—————

My Rumbles with Anxiety

"The way of out of fear isn't safety. It is freedom."
– Martha Beck

I t was November 24, 1963, two days after President John F. Kennedy was killed. I was born one month early. The whole world was in mourning. I came in with an incredible urgency, like the world was on fire and I had better hurry up and help save it. I always felt late, and like things were moving too darn slow. Growing up in a family with alcoholism rampant on both sides was challenging, I felt invisible and unimportant. I learned how to put my radar on and predict my next move to keep everyone OK. I chose to become the caretaker of my parents' marriage, which included being my mother's confidante, in order to feel seen and valuable. Knowing too much just added to my anxiety. I became a little adult fast. My uninvited guest was there from the beginning, I suppose. It's intention, I believe, was to help me survive.

As a child, the world felt scary. People seemed unhappy and clueless. My mom had significant health issues when I was young, so she wanted me to grow up as soon as possible. I did too. I figured the more grown-up I could be, the more control I would have. It made perfect sense to me.

My anxiety became overwhelming. I found a new way to cope by being highly critical of myself, to the point of self-loathing. By the time I was in 7th grade, I hated every single part of my body. I never felt good enough. Perfection was unreachable, but it felt like the answer to being safe and secure in the world. At age 12, I was chased by two adult men in a car while I was walking home from school one day. They didn't catch me, but I felt utterly terrified and exposed, more than I already was. Now my radar was on literally all the time.

By my teenage years, my anxiety had bunked up with depression, and I felt suicidal often. Back then, you just silently suffered. No one had heard of treatment. I began experimenting with substances the way I saw my family cope, numbing myself more than I already did with food. I also became a people-pleaser and chameleon on top of being a perfectionist. It is how I "did" school, relationships, friendships, everything. "Do better. Be more," I said to myself. I would push myself all the time, while inside I felt like a failure. I didn't even realize I was living with anxiety. I thought everyone was like this.

Looking back through my life, I see how certain teachers and spiritual traditions came across my path starting in my twenties that guided me through my hard times and moved me along toward growth and healing. They were such blessings. They kept me evolving in the face of despair and suffering.

By the time I was finishing college, I felt quite anxious about my future. My relationships were still anxiety-provoking and unstable. At age 23, I connected with Native American traditions for three years, which I felt naturally akin to. I was fortunate to study *The Sweet Medicine Sundance Teachings of the Chuluaqui-Quodoushka,* by Harley Swiftdeer Reagan, with my teacher Dr. Liz Chandra(1). I learned a new respect for my body, sexuality, and Mother Earth. I was taught the rituals of pipe ceremony, sweat lodge purification, and other practices. This was the beginning of my deeper learning about the meaning of life, which soothed my anxiety and connected me more with myself.

Within a few years I met Don Miguel Ruiz, a teacher of the *Toltec tradition* who later wrote *The Four Agreements*(2). I was guided to apprentice with Don Miguel Ruiz, for the next eight years. I understood more about humanity's pain and suffering and what I could do about it. I began to dismantle my own wounding inner critic. I could stop judging myself and others so harshly, for the first time ever. This had a very positive impact on my anxiety.

In my early thirties, I was finishing grad school and teaching the Toltec *path*. I had made some progress with my sense of self and my anxiety was better. Then I got married and had kids at 35 years old. Anxiety quickly erupted. My marriage was a disaster. My husband got lost in alcohol and was emotionally abusive. I was treading water. I ended up with Perinatal Mood and Anxiety Disorder during both pregnancies and postpartum periods. It was the most painful experience of my life. Being a mother felt too important to screw up. I was a wreck. And being a wreck when you have two little babies to care for was absolute torture. My capacity to manage life was missing in action.

I luckily found Postpartum Support International (PSI) on the internet when my midwives and doctors were not informed enough to be helpful. PSI helps families understand what mood and anxiety issues mothers can have and how to recover(3). They said I had to ask for help if I wanted to get well. This was problematic, because I had learned to rarely ask for anything. Yet learning this one act humbled me and saved my life. I had to care for and value myself in a whole new way. Like the airplane safety procedure message, "Put your own oxygen mask on before helping your child," this became my hardest accomplishment and my personal mantra for many years. I became passionate about keeping other moms from suffering endlessly and devoted 12 years to educating health practitioners and treating families with PMADs.

As a part of my practice of asking and receiving more help, I entered psychotherapy and later coaching. I worked my tail off for many years. This helped me survive negotiating my divorce and our child custody issues, after my marriage fell apart a short time later. My anxiety skyrocketed. I felt terrified about my kid's safety and my ability to be a single parent of two kid with no help. I knew I needed more support. I started to go to Al-Anon programs for the first time(4). I had never learned so much about alcoholism and how it affects those around it. It helped me put the pieces of my struggles and anxieties together in a new way that was very clarifying. I created a spiritual connection that served me well through those terrifying court battle years. I grew up a lot. I could keep seeing how my anxiety was just a part of me, not a ruler of me.

Years later, I started taking Kundalini yoga classes again after 20 years to continue improving my own self-care. It was wonderfully healing for me to be in a community again, when I felt so personally isolated. Within a few years, I decided to go through teacher training at Yoga Santa Fe with Kirn and GC Khalsa(4,5). It was intense and powerful. I cleared out more fear and anxiety and was feeling more connected with myself. I established a meditation discipline that I had always wished for. I taught classes for a year and facilitated some retreats. I felt like I was on my way to the life I had always imagined.

Then a year later, I got ovarian cancer. I thought "Why now?" I had made it through so much. I finally ate well, I exercised, I took care of myself, and I was nicer to myself than ever before. I even meditated, for Goddess' sake! This wasn't supposed to happen. After the surgery, I argued with myself and the doctors' orders of treatment. I struggled to control the outcome and do it my way as my old strategy. All my old fears resurfaced. I realized this was my next opportunity to let go even more of my old friend, anxiety and control, as my way to cope. I asked for help in letting go and trusting in a new way. I surrendered deeply into my heart and listened to my inner wisdom for the best treatment path for me. It wasn't about finding the "right way" for me, it was about choosing a way for me to let go and trust the process. And by the gift of grace, I came through it. I felt like I woke up again to how amazing, beautiful, and luscious life is. I wanted to keep that perspective.

I learned how my greatest ally was my body, that had carried me through everything in spite of myself.

Over the next few years, I felt compelled to deepen my embodiment practices even more. I was pulled to learn more of this body-based spirituality that I had briefly studied 30 years before. I had become aware of how disembodied I had become. I began training in Tantra Kriya yoga with Richard and Antoinette of Tantra Heart(6). Essentially, it is about the body's systems of energy, consciousness, and spirituality. In that same year, I had the good fortune to also learn Divine Feminine embodiment practices with Chameli Ardagh of Awakening Women(7). These paths greatly empowered my re-connection with my own body, mind, emotions, sexuality, and spirit. My anxiety became easier to name, know, and diffuse.

Then I serendipitously found Reggie Ray and his body-based meditation of Tibetan Buddhism, which he calls the Somatic Meditation of Pure Awareness(9). I realized that I had been studying this lineage of Trungpa Rinpoche already, with Pema Chodron, another student of his who I fell in love with ten years prior(8). This embodiment practice was the step towards deeper somatic work I had been asking for. It just amazes me how when we ask for guidance, it may cross our paths a few times before we see it or are ready for it. I know my anxiety even more now and know how to use it to my advantage in life. It keeps opening me to possibilities to get out in the world and serve more women.

I acknowledge the blessings of these traditions and teachings that have guided me through my life struggles. This Fear-Less program comes from all of my steps and experiences. We all have our own life paths of struggles and blessings to honor. I do not claim that these teachings are the only way, and they have made an incredible difference for me and my clients over the past 30 years, so I offer them from this place. Take what works and leave the rest. In the past, I was always open to try new things because I truly felt I could not survive staying where I was. I had nothing to lose. Perhaps that is true for you as well. May you benefit from your experiences with this program.

"When one has nothing to lose, one becomes courageous."
– Carlos Castaneda

CHAPTER 3

The Fear-Less Path

"The greatest mistake we make is living in constant fear
that we will make one."
– Maxwell

When anxiety is messing with you and your life, you just want it gone. You want to be yourself again. You want to be able to handle what life throws at you and not get paralyzed with anxiety attacks. You want to have the energy to do what you want. You want to be able to sleep through the night. You want to feel comfortable in your body. You want to get out in the world and do what you feel inspired to do. You just want anxiety to leave you alone!

This book was designed to teach you how to make all of that happen. It was created for women just like you and me who want a life without anxiety. It is about changing our old default patterns in our brains and bodies so we can be in charge. We all have what we need inside of us, but we don't always know how to access it and use it wisely. Our minds, bodies, and spirits are these amazing intricate systems that work together in powerful ways. We can either unconsciously be hurting ourselves with our default habits or we can be conscious and use our mind, body, and spirit to grow, heal, evolve, and become our best self.

In this approach, we learn to use these systems to our advantage. The more we can start being who we truly are without anxiety running us, the more our lives can change dramatically. I think of it as looking through fresh eyes at ourselves and the world. We see things we never noticed before. We start to recognize what is possible.

The Fear-Less Approach

Let's take a look at how this Fear-Less approach is laid out. It was created specifically for women, which makes this a unique anxiety program that empowers the feminine. We utilize three principle archetypes of woman – the Queen, the Heroine, and the Goddess – to guide us in identifying different parts of ourselves we can draw on to defeat anxiety. In this program, these archetypes are associated with the three essential human dimensions: The Mind, the Body, and the Spirit. Even though we are looking at the human dimensions as separate entities for simplicity, keep in mind that they are always interactive and interdependent.

Another distinguishing characteristic of this program is primary role of the Body. I have found that most of the modalities that work with anxiety are far more effective when we relate them back to the dimension of the Body. The act of perceiving our experiences through the Body is the missing link in many anxiety theories and practices. This is what makes this particular program so dynamic and impactful, standing out from many others, in my experience.

In Part Two, we focus on the Queen domain. The Queen represents the Mind in this path. The Queen is the aspect of woman that is solid, regal, and mature. She is powerful in and of herself, as a woman. She helps reconnect us with our personal power so we can put anxiety in its place. In the first Chapter of the Queen, Worth, we look at the role of our inner critic and the fear stories that keep our anxiety going. Then we move into the Dignity chapter to learn about our self-regard, and self-responsibility and their relationship with our anxiety. In the last Queen chapter, Sovereignty, we explore our beliefs to see if they align with what we truly want or if they support our anxiety to keep running us.

In Part Three, we move into the Heroine Principle's territory. The Heroine represents our feminine daring, strength, and courage, as the Body aspect. She is our "inner spiritual warrior," our powerful, embodied, feminine side who shows up and does what it takes to reclaim our lives from anxiety. Here our Body is our greatest ally. Our culture has, on the contrary, taught us to mistreat our bodies as objects and even hate them. This is a real problem when our greatest ally is our most hated enemy. It leads to anxiety in a multitude of ways.

Reverence is the first quality of the Body we practice. We look at the consequences of how lost and disconnected from our bodies we have become. We learn about the power of embodiment and breath in aiding us with our anxiety. The second quality of the Body is Wisdom. We discuss the importance of emotional intelligence and gaining awareness of the feelings and sensations in our body. Once we have laid key groundwork for feelings and body awareness, we focus on releasing old wounds with the Coming Home process.

In Part Four, we explore the Goddess Principle. The Goddess represents our Spiritual domain, our Divine Self. The Goddess is the face of our developed Feminine Consciousness, our inner knowing, intuition, and connection with the living world around us. In this approach, remember that the path of spiritual connection is through the Body. We always stay embodied to access and experience our higher consciousness within us, not outside of us.

The first quality of the Spirit Domain is Gratitude. In this chapter, we cover the spiritual and physiological effects of gratitude and how they apply in transforming anxiety. In the next Chapter, on Loving–Kindness, we learn the essence of living with care and consciousness. We discuss the relevant teachings that speak to the importance of impeccability with our words and actions. This directly applies to life with less anxiety.

The last quality of Spirit we delve into is Divine Connection. This chapter speaks to how we personally develop and attune to our divine connection. It is about the golden thread that connects us with Spirit, allowing us to perceive the interconnection of all things. This is where we can cultivate our sense of empowerment and personal freedom, helping us see the bigger picture of life. It is a necessary piece of being our best selves in the face of anxiety.

The Best Way to Apply This Book

Now let's talk about how this book can support you the most. Once you have started reading this book, know that it's already changing you. It's like when you know you are going to get a new haircut and it changes the way you feel about yourself, even before it happens. The mind is already moving toward that moment. Your perception is already preparing for the change. Your intent, your heart, your spirit are already seeing your future. So you want to take your time and take it all in. This is like a gorgeous, long road trip, not a race. You want to catch the scenery, meet the people, and try the food. Read it and enjoy it. Let it percolate inside you. Try the practices at your own pace. This is not an academic book that has a test at the end. What matters here is reading, digesting, and practicing this approach. The more you practice, the more you absorb the powerful vitamins and nutrients of this Fear-Less path. The knowledge comes by experiencing what happens within you. Knowledge is only as important as it provides a context for us to live, learn, and grow in. Your experience is what matters the most. This path is about you showing up and living with new awareness of yourself, which will empower you to live a life without anxiety.

"Tell me, what is it you plan to do with
your one wild and precious life?"
– Mary Oliver

PART TWO:

The Queen

"It's believing in those dreams and facing our fears head on that allows us to live beyond our limits."

– Amy Purdy

CHAPTER 4

The Mind

"The purpose of life as a woman is to ascend
to the throne and rule with heart."
– Marianne Williamson

The Queen archetype is the beautiful ruler of our Mind. She represents our potential to make our minds one of our greatest assets, if we take our power back from fear. The Queen is the reflection of how we see ourselves and our own sense of personal power. She reveals how we feel about being a woman, which depends greatly on the environment we grow up in. Women's lives have always been shaped by the cultural views of the acceptable female roles of the times, acknowledges Jean Shiboda Bolen(1). Today, in the face of the failing patriarchal constructs, the world is in dire need of the return of feminine principles to bring things back to into balance.

Marianne Williamson, in her book *A Woman's Worth,* proclaims, "Womanhood is being recast, and we're pregnant, en masse, giving birth to our own redemption." The Queen archetype reconnects us with our inherent goodness and feminine strength as women. Many of us may have never connected with the Queen aspect inside of us before. We have unknowingly stayed stuck in our young Princess archetype, who is devoted to pleasing her daddy and other men in her life, to feel approved of. We don't even know who we are or what we want because we are so focused on caring for others. This is no longer serving anyone truly.

Our beliefs impact how we see the world, how we feel, and how we respond to life's circumstances. Our anxiety can reinforce beliefs like *life is scary* and *problems lurk at every corner.* We need to be the Queen of our Mind to be in charge of what we believe, instead of being victimized by our fearful beliefs. We will discuss the essential qualities we need to develop to take back dominion of our minds.

I remember after my divorce, 17 years ago, a friend of mine did a tarot reading for me and said, "You are going to be fine, eventually. You will be the queen of your castle." At the time, I felt more like a slave to the bills, single-parenting my kids, working on my issues, and building my practice. I did not feel like a queen at all. But that image, or we can say the energy of the archetype, stayed with me in the back of my mind. Many years later, I bought a new house. When I was in my new bedroom with incredible space, views, walk-in closet, and everything I had always wanted, I suddenly thought "I am the Queen of my castle now!" I had manifested this physical reflection of finally treating myself as a Queen. I can see how I kept opening my beliefs to what was possible despite my current challenges. We can all learn how to do this.

In the rest of Part Two, we focus on the qualities that are essential for us cultivate in the face of anxiety. First, we will address Worth, as the first step towards developing our Queen self and learn about our ego mind. We will work with our self-respect in the chapter on Dignity. Then we use that foundation to reclaim our personal authority in the Sovereignty chapter. It is time to rule, Queens.

CHAPTER 5

Worth

"We cannot solve our problems with the same thinking
that we used when we created them."
– Albert Einstein

To be the Queen, one must know one's own Worth. Self-Worth is the sense of one's own value as a human being. Here it also relates to our worth to be in charge of our own minds.

The first accomplice to our anxiety that we need to learn about is the Inner Parent part of our Ego Mind. This is the voice in our heads that comes from our parents, grandparents, teachers, or anyone who represents authority. It most often is a critical voice, not a nurturing voice. It is born out of our early personality development and biological need to please and be approved of and loved so we can survive. We all learn quickly how to get love in the "acceptable" way our family and culture taught us. This is what Toltec tradition calls our "domestication:" how we learn the unspoken rules of our family and culture to fit in. This Inner Parent births our Inner Critic, who becomes a large part of our anxiety.

The Inner Critic

This Inner Critic (IC) is usually the loudest voice in our head and the first on the scene. It "harbors secret self-condemnation and guilt for things it has done or failed to do(1)." This part of our ego carries deep shame and cannot fully accept or give forgiveness or love as a result. It continually criticizes, compares, and blames others and ourselves in an effort to survive. It is not a happy-camper part of us at all. It only knows how to rehash the past and fantasize about the future without taking action to do anything differently. It is the stuck part of us.

The IC's original motivations are to save us from external shame, blame, punishment, and embarrassment when we are young. However, it ends up becoming the perpetrator of these emotions in its efforts to "protect us," and causes anxiety in the process. We begin to believe we need it to keep us on track, that without it, we would never get off the couch. It tells us all kinds of stories of failure that say if we don't do what it says, we will always be failures. This is most painful part of the IC; when it tells us we are worthless unless we accomplish this, that, and the other thing. It is so caught up in the patriarchal view of a person's value being based on what they achieve that we can be very wounded when we accept its distortions as truth. It can be mean, hurtful, discounting, unreasonable, hyper-critical, and rude. This often leads to us to being self-loathing and self-destructive in an effort to mitigate our anxiety while it is the behavior that actually perpetuates it. The Fear-Less Path will teach us how to be aware of and how to disempower our IC and its affliction.

Now pause a moment and think about your own IC. This is where we get to recognize how our family lineage can affect the way we think, emote, and see the world. Our family IC gets handed down generations and generations – unless we retrain it. You got this, my Queen.

Practice #1: Shadowing Your Inner Critic

This is a practice of observing. We put our attention to learning all we can about our Inner Critic. You can study it from afar or interview it up close. You are like an investigative journalist, trying to find out all you can about it. In Toltec tradition, this is called stalking. Your objective is to identify where you are wasting energy that could be used for new growth and freedom from past mental habits. Watch and learn your thinking patterns, then question and interrupt them. Let's take a minute to think about your own Inner Critic. Get some paper out and answer these questions, taking all the time you need.

How is your IC like your mom's or dad's voice? When does it show up the most? When is it the meanest? And when is it relatively quiet? When are you immune to its ramblings? Why do you think that is?

When are you most susceptible and totally wrung out by it? How long has this IC version been around? How does it hurt you?

What is it actually afraid about? Is it right to be worried, or is it full of it? Is it ever helpful, or is it just a control freak? What does your IC really want from you?

It can be helpful to notice if some of the answers above spark your anxiety. In fact, let's have you go through and answer the same questions as if you were interviewing your anxiety now. Take another five or ten minutes. Breathe. Stay present. With this practice, you increase your observation and awareness skills. Once you learn more about your IC and your anxiety, you can become smarter about how and when you indulge them and when you can shift your attention away from them and stop strengthening them. You get to see that the IC is just a part of you, not in charge of you.

My sweet client Sarah, who is 45 and married, is working on her chronic anxiety. She had been in a dysfunctional, emotionally abusive family growing up, and her romantic relationships followed that pattern as well. She never feels good enough in herself and puts everyone else first and suffers greatly as a result. Her anxiety has her convinced there is no way out. She is studying her IC. As she engages in valuing herself more and putting herself first, things are really starting to shift. She is speaking up and setting boundaries, despite her husband's discomfort and anger. She is no longer indulging her IC, and instead is becoming the Queen of her life – in charge, without worry overruling her.

Sometimes, we literally have to fight for the right to reclaim our worth, because as women, we have been fooled into believing that we don't have value. The misogynistic patriarchy has had us believing we are less than men for hundreds of years.

We need to remember that our worth is inherent – it is with us when we are born and when we die. Our merit is not based on achievement, looks, or character. It is a given. It is always there, whether we choose to see it or not. So how can we stay connected with this truth of our inherent virtue and value? We need to strengthen a different part of our mind called the Observer Self, or our Witness. The Witness is a fundamental skill to cultivate on this Fear-Less Path.

Your Witness Perspective

The Witness Self is also called the Neutral Mind in yoga tradition. The Witness Self lives outside of the ego and the duality of good and bad. This part can observe us, our minds, our bodies, and our thoughts, but it never judges us. It simply watches and assesses from an instinctual awareness. When we develop our Witness perspective, we can learn to disengage from our ego. We can discern which thoughts and beliefs will empower us and which we will suppress us. This is a necessary skill-set as we hone in on responding instead of reacting to our anxiety's fear stories.

We must first be conscious of our body to connect with our Witness Self. We begin with our physical awareness and then notice our thinking mind. We start taking inventory of the fear stories we tell ourselves. Anxiety is a state of mind that impacts our thinking and then triggers our nervous system to start revving up for a fight, flight, or freeze situation – whether the threat is real or not. We want to catch these fears when they are just showing up, before they take over our nervous system. We want to be able to identify when we are at a level 1 on a scale of 1-10 of a fear reaction, before we reach a level 5 or 8. We can do this with our Witness.

When we are in our Witness perspective, we can more easily stay connected to our self-worth. In our fear stories, which live in our ego mind, we lose our sense of self-worth. Many fear stories may come from our experiences in our childhoods, when we did not have the tools to deal with them. We simply had to make quick assessments and decisions like, "Let's avoid that in the future." Consequently, when we get anxious as adults, we are often stuck in our younger selves and their immature beliefs about the world like "It's all my fault." Our fear stories also love to project the past onto to the future with worst-case scenarios, even if they are pretty unlikely or even irrational. Our ego, which lives in fear, assumes the worst in the present based on the past. The "What if?" scenarios wipe out the moment completely. When we can identify and reframe our fear stories with our Witness, then we have a choice of how to respond to them in the moment instead of being governed by our anxiety.

Theresa, a 35-year-old amazing school teacher, suffers with fear and constant tension. When she began working with her Witness, she was finding it difficult to discern between it and her ego. She practices observing herself, and suddenly the ego takes over and starts being critical with her. Now she uses a breathing practice, with her ego mind focusing on counting the pace of the breath, while her Witness can experience what is present. This is helping her get better at distinguishing between them. She is connecting with her Witness faster and easier and keeping the ego out of the way longer, each time we meet. As a result, she feels calmer and less distressed.

Practice #2: Soothing Our Fear Stories

To practice being in your Witness, you must be present and on board in your body. This means feeling the ground beneath you and being conscious of your breath. Begin with 3-10 deep belly breaths with your lower belly filling out on the inhale and receding on the exhale. Begin observing your fear stories from the most recent anxiety occurrences. What would happen if you could notice the fear mindset objectively versus reacting to it right away as if it were coming true? Imagine stepping back and noticing what is happening in your mind-body awareness. See if you can observe your fear, acknowledge its assumptions rather than letting it overtake you. You can even welcome its opinion and say to yourself, "Here is my fear telling me this story." When you can recognize fear's story as just a story and not the truth, you can then allow it to pass through without attaching to it. In her book, *Hope and Help for your Nerves*, Claire Weekes calls this observing and acknowledging action "floating." When you are floating, your mind can be aware of the thoughts, stories, and sensations of fear without getting stuck in them. You can continue doing what you planned to do while floating through the sensations of the anxiety. I also offer the imagery that you are the ocean, vast and wide, and the anxiety and life's ups and downs are but little waves on your surface, not able to disrupt the depths of the ocean's floor.

Some people benefit from actively soothing their fear stories. As the adult conscious part of yourself, you can choose to pacify the fearful part of you through acknowledging it and then consoling it rather than letting it run the show. You can say, "I see that you're scared. It's OK. Nothing is wrong." Try this out. See what happens and how your body responds. In this way, you are meeting your fear. You are not ignoring it, believing it, or giving it power. You are paying attention to what is showing up. This can become a potent tool when you use it regularly.

When 42-year-old professional business woman, Christie, first started working with me, her fear stories took her completely over when they came, especially at work. She practices noticing the fear's patterns, sensations and signs in order to catch it earlier before it is at a 10 on a scale of 0-10. She is becoming more observant of her thoughts that change. When she spots her fearful thinking at a 3 and moderates it, then she can float through the experience and stay on task. Some people learn this process by attending to their thoughts, and others can notice it more in their bodies' sensations. Christie is understanding how to stop getting hooked by her fear patterns so she can keep on task at work. Soon Christie and I will explore the fear's meaning.

When we are first working with our anxiety, our nerves and reactions are often overwrought, and it isn't necessary to know what is triggering the fear. If you can recognize the fear story, that's great. If not, don't worry about it. Just work with the accepting the anxiety and floating with it. Keep relaxing the body as much as possible. Later, when your nerves are calmer and your capacity to not get hooked by the fear is stronger, you can begin to identify triggers and related emotions. We cover this more in later chapters.

Self-Forgiveness Supports Your Self-Worth

As we learn more about our Inner Critic and our fear stories, we naturally can be more in touch with our virtue, our goodness. Another way we support our sense of self and clear the path to our worthiness is through self-forgiveness. Forgiveness is a practice of compassion and mercy with ourselves for believing our fears and IC's lies about who we are. We can see how it hurts us when we believe them. Past life events and traumas, of course, contribute to the fears, but right now we are focusing on the importance of living in the present time, where we are enough and doing the best we can. We forgive, out of generosity, kindness and love for ourselves, to counterbalance the old shame and blame that are part of those fear stories. This might be difficult at first but be the Queen and do the best you can.

Practice #3: Mirror-Work for Forgiveness

This is a self-forgiveness practice to reclaim your self-worth. Stand before a mirror that is small enough to show your face only. Know that using a mirror to give your internal critic room to beat you up and degrade you is no longer acceptable. Focus only on our eyes. Look beyond the physical eyes for the eyes of your soul. Talk from ownership about your self-judgment and say, "Please forgive me for believing I am unworthy. I value, love, and accept you." Say it multiple times until you show up. Receive the message in your mind, body, and spirit. Allow the feelings and tears to come. Release the shame and pain of the many years of criticalness, judgment, and self-rejection. This is most powerful when used as a daily practice for a minimum of three weeks. Stay with it and it will become one the most powerful tools to reset yourself in your tool-bag, when you get off kilter and full of judgment and fear.

Mary Jo, who is age 49, and a dedicated family law attorney, coaches with me for her anxiety attacks that are increasingly debilitating her. She is married, has two young kids and her own business. Her anxiety stops her world from working. We identify early on that she is carrying a ton of past shame and self-judgment. She is highly motivated so I taught her about mirror-work. She is embarrassed and shameful at first, no surprise. I let her know that is part of it, feeling all those painful feelings and to hang in there and hold onto the forgiveness and acceptance. She recently shared with me that she is feeling less shameful and she is being kinder to herself without really "working hard on it". I told her this is the point-to stop working it so hard-and practice how to be accepting with herself wherever she is. Mirror-work can feel like a simple process, but it's power is deep and profound.

We will learn in later chapters how to face old wounds and work with other modalities of forgiveness. For now, we want to start inviting the idea of forgiving ourselves from a simple awareness that we are always doing our best. When we can do better, we usually do. I always think of my client Lacy, who has such amazing results in supporting her self-worth with this basic concept of accepting that she is doing her best. She embraced the 'I am good enough" concept. She calls this her "super-power" now because she can derail her Inner Critic so well with this one modality.

When we disempower our judgments and fears and begin forgiving ourselves, we are clearing the path for reclaiming our Self-Worth. It's analogous to pushing the clouds away so we can feel the sun's rays on our face. Our mind needs to be a clear blue sky so that the sun, our Soul, can shine through us, unobstructed. This prepares us for developing our next necessary quality, our Dignity as the Queen.

Main Messages:

1. Our Queen can control the Inner Critic by learning all about it and being more aware.
2. When we engage our Witness, we can keep our fear stories from driving us.
3. Our Self-Worth never leaves us, ever.

Additional Tools of Discovery

1. Stand as a Queen. Find your regular posture and observe your thoughts about yourself. Now stand tall and regal like a Queen for 5 minutes. Posture affects our thoughts, emotions, and resilience(2). Emanate your Queen-ness as if you are standing before the royal court. Breathe, feel your energy as Queen, your thoughts and feelings. Notice how you feel about yourself. How powerful do you feel? Is your anxiety around? Embody all the awareness you have right now. Then write it down, or find a picture to reflect what that felt like. Put it up somewhere you can see it every day to remind you.
2. Affirmations. Try these, or use your own. Say them 3-4 times per day for 90 days.

"I am noticing and dismissing my Inner Critic more each day."

"I am worthy and valuable always."

"I can observe and float past my fears."

CHAPTER 6

―――――――

Dignity

"A woman in harmony with her spirit is like a river flowing
She goes where she will without pretense and arrives at her
destination prepared to be herself
And only herself."
– Maya Angelou

This chapter focuses on the reconstruction of our self-regard, care, and responsibility as the Queen. Cultivating our respect for the feminine aspects of ourselves is crucial. The role of feminine dignity has been defaced by our patriarchal culture, therefore we must recall the ancient esteem and honor of the feminine deep within our souls. This includes having respect for other women as well. Having been taught by our culture to compete with and vilify each other in exchange for feeling secure, better than, and more valuable about ourselves, we have cut off our noses to spite our faces. The sisterhood of women, full of love and support for one another, is our birthright as women. It is a beautiful secret garden that can deeply nourish and feed our souls. Yet, we have learned to not want it, to devalue it, and to look to serve men instead, for our personal worth and approval. This is a monumental loss that must be recovered.

The Honor of Self-Responsibility

When we choose to restore our sense of self-dignity as the Queen, it means we take complete responsibility for ourselves now. We cannot do that if we are attached to being a victim in our lives. Being in a victim role keeps us powerless and at the mercy of other people and their choices. Then we have no authority of our lives and it is wretched. Research validates that when we feel that we have no control over ourselves and our lives, we will have significantly increased anxiety and decreased sense of well-being[1,2].

We all have been victimized at some point in our lives, when we had no way to stop something awful from happening to us. It is a tragic common experience. When this happens, it is our personal duty to get support to process the experience the best we can. When we can take care of ourselves and choose to learn from it, we can move forward with our sense of self intact. When we don't do this, we can get stuck and mistakenly believe we will never get past it or be capable in ourselves again. We have lost connection with our experience as a powerful human. This is an unbearable story that ruins lives. We all have one thing we can be in charge of, and that is how we respond to life, in all its joys and hardships. Many of us may not know this because we have never been taught. It is OK, my Queen. You got this.

We start with Self-Respect, which means having regard for the dignity of one's character. It means caring about yourself. As young girls, we are taught to be "ladylike," which means we learn to sacrifice ourselves to care for everyone else's needs, even at our own expense. Even in 2017, this continues to be the unconscious expectation of men, society, and even ourselves. It is a deep disregard for women as individuals with passions and purposes of their own. We are the ones who can change that.

We can begin learning self-respect by recognizing that taking care of ourselves truly serves people in our lives far better than living out of obligation, fear of being rejected, and martyrdom. When we live to please others in exchange for feeling OK and approved of, it doesn't really meet our needs. It eventually leads to what I call "a people-pleaser's tornado of resentment." As people-pleasers, we secretly think that if we are there for others, they will be there for us. This generally does not happen. We have already taught people that we are the ones who will bend over backwards for them. In the Toltec tradition, we learn how important it is to never go against ourselves or each other, as this drains our personal energy and power. The Four Agreements show us that the way to care for ourselves is to honor and respect ourselves by stopping our judging, assuming, and taking things personally. We can never feel truly loved, seen, and accepted as a people-pleaser. We must get it first from ourselves. This happens when we take responsibility for our self-respect and care.

Winny, age 60, is a sweet retired school teacher. She has never learned to respect herself, because she was treated horribly by her mother as a child. She gets upset when her husband disregards her, but she also tolerates it, unconsciously feeling that she doesn't deserve better. As she develops her own self-respect in our work together, she is finding that her husband and other people seem to be behaving with more kindness and regard for her. She is stunned. This isn't magic, it is the mirror of life. How we treat ourselves on the inside reflects in how others treat us on the outside.

Knowing Your Boundaries

Another way we can respect ourselves is by learning to be responsible for ourselves by understanding our own boundaries. Boundaries are a natural sense of identity that separates us from each other as individuals. We can often sense our boundaries more than we know them concretely. For example, when someone stands too close to your personal space and you start to feel uncomfortable, that is a way of sensing that someone has crossed your spatial boundaries. Once you know that, you can ask people to step back and say, "Thank you, that works better for me." Other boundaries are emotional. For example, some people do not mind sarcasm, and others are uncomfortable and sensitive to it. Neither is right or wrong, they are simply personality differences and comfort levels. Speaking up and letting people know, "I don't care for sarcasm, thank you," is essential in having our own backs. We always have the right to ask for what we need. We may or may not receive what we are requesting from others, but it is still important that we speak up and communicate it. When people cannot give us what we request, we still have choices. For example, once when I was at a table with friends who were talking loud and my ears were hurting, I asked them if they were willing to talk quieter. They looked at me funny and blew me off. So, I chose to get up and go sit somewhere else. My needs are my responsibility. I was proud of myself for standing up for myself and for not judging myself or them as wrong. Boundaries take time to master, we will always be developing them.

There are also sexual boundaries and mental boundaries of what are acceptable ways of being touched or treated. Everyone is different. We need to acknowledge and assert our limits as part of self-responsibility, despite what our families, our bosses, or the bullies in our lives may say about it. It is how we teach people who we are, what we like, and what we absolutely do not put up with. We teach people how they need to treat us. If we do not know what those limits are for ourselves because we have been people-pleasers most of our lives, then this will take some practice to get good at it. And this is the perfect time. Because not knowing your limits and boundaries is a big part of anxiety.

Nina is a friendly young mom of two small children who is highly stressed and anxious. She struggles with a belief that, for her to be loving and loved, she needs to be pleasing all the time. She confuses love with having no boundaries. Despite her inner conflict, she is practicing setting a few limits at home. It has not been smooth and easy. Her kids and her husband are adjusting. She is hanging in there despite their resistances. She realizes how angry she feels deep inside when she is not taking care of herself as well as she does her family. She is reinforcing her self-respect in herself every time she has a boundary she sticks up for. She is experiencing her Dignity. I doubt she will ever look back. It's nearly impossible once you have excavated your Queen

Practice #1: Identifying Your Boundaries

Start being aware of your response to your environments and what is irritating, stimulating, or annoying to you. There are probably some boundaries there that you are unaware of that you need to set. Notice when people are demanding things of you. What are you thinking and feeling? What would you like to say to them, and what do you end up saying instead? Think about what boundaries you would want in place next time this happens. Having personal limits support us in being calmer, healthier, more efficient, and happier. They also stop us from pushing ourselves too hard and too far. For example, learning to take breaks at work to reboot your mind and body so you can come back and get the job done with less stress is a powerful example of boundaries. Practicing listening to your inner wisdom and intuition is important as well, instead of being run by your ego mind that says "keep going," which you know leads to burnout, tension, and anxiety.

Take a moment now and think of some basic boundaries you know you need to work on. Write them down for the different areas of your life, for example: parenting, marriage, work, friendships, and health. Notice where you need the most focus for developing your personal self-regard and responsibility. Once you realize that boundaries are all about loving yourself, you will feel less guilty about having and asserting them. The world would be a much happier place if everyone knew and used their boundaries. And for sure, people would have much less anxiety.

The Loving Respect of Self-Care

Another form of dignity is recognizing our self-responsibility every day through self-care. Staying mindful and devoted to our own care and wellbeing in all the small nurturing, mindful ways is key, especially in the face of anxiety. Self-care starves anxiety. Self-care asks that we keep ourselves at the top of our to-do list all the time, recognizing that if we are fed, attended to, well-rested, exercised, meditated, listened to, loved, and appreciated, then we are more equipped to go out in the world and share your gifts. And when we do show up for others, our cups are full and overflowing. We are nurtured from the inside-out. We behave like a people who love ourselves, even if we don't completely believe it yet on the inside.

Betty, age 66, is a dedicated and anxious woman, who grew up in New Mexico with all the old cultural traditions handed down to her by her mother. She serves everyone else first, and I mean the entire extended family. She never gives herself a break. She is so caught up being enough for her mother, who criticizes her regularly, that anxiety is a constant presence for Betty. All her denied needs, feelings, and wants live inside her anxiety. She came to see me again after her mother and husband died. Betty needed to figure out how she can put herself first, even with it bringing up her guilt. It her takes her some time and practice to build up her boundaries and self-care practices to be part of her daily routine. She considers herself to be freer now than she has ever felt in her lifetime. Her anxiety and people-pleasing are less able to run her for very long. Her true sense of Dignity is growing present and more intact.

Practice #2: Daily Self-Care

Here is a basic formula for daily self-care. Add to it or modify it. Find what helps you the most, then do it regularly, because that is the name of the game with self-care. Routines are a structure to help your new behaviors become habits. If you do a new behavior daily for 90 days, it has the most chance to survive your ego's resistance and become part of your daily life.

1. Self-Time. Living in a busy world, we all need different degrees of alone time. This is in addition to couple time and family time. Self-time is the foundation for being more present and available when we do spend time with others. If your own cup is empty, how can you nurture these relationships?

2. Mindfulness in Nature: Practice moments of focused awareness without doing anything. I recommend sitting in nature with no phone. Listen to the sounds, feel the air, notice your breath, and see the beauty around you. Time in nature has been proven to positively affect your health, well-being, and social interaction(3). Take a good 5-10 minutes, when possible.

3. Conscious Breathing: Observe your breath and body while you count the pace of the breath. Slowly begin to match the inhale and exhale pace. Notice how calm

your nervous system is after just a few minutes. Practice twice a day for 3-5 minutes.

4. Daily Grounding: Breathing with awareness of your body helps you to be more present in your whole body, instead of being a head walking around. Your Earth connection also promotes your resilience to stress and supports your wellbeing(4). Take 10 minutes with your bare feet on the actual surface of dirt, water, or sand. Allow the release of stress and the refill of good energy to happen simply.

5. Gratitude: Gratitude as a daily practice increases our sense of happiness and openness to social support(5). Keep a gratitude journal, or just start your day with acknowledgment of something you are grateful for. Feel it come into your heart. Notice how it can literally change the sensations, attitude, and mood in your mind and body.

6. Disconnect: Disconnect from all screens for a least an hour a day before sleep. And one day a week if possible, be completely screen-free. The quiet and space from technology alone are highly beneficial for your mental and physical health(6). It's easy to think we are getting rest when we watch TV, but it's not the same mental release as when we rest in the backyard and watch the stars or sit on the porch. Notice.

7. Sleep: Get at least 7-8 hours of sleep every night. Sleep is the most undervalued, essential aspect of self-care in our culture. If you want to be efficient, get sleep. If you

want to be calm, get sleep. If you want to have a leg up on anxiety, get sleep.

8. Positive Acknowledgment: Give yourself three positive acknowledgments for every negative comment that comes from your mind. Purposely notice the positive experiences, thoughts, and moods more often, instead of letting our default ego scan only for the negative all the time. Practice only sharing with others about the positive experiences for a week and see what happens.

When we become friends with our self-care and boundaries, they no longer require so much effort. They become part of self-love and respect in a way that feels honorable. And of course, it helps us get better at transforming our anxiety.

Main Messages:

1. Dignity comes with our Queen's Self-Regard and Self-Responsibility.
2. Having Dignity means we identify and set our boundaries to respect ourselves.
3. Self-care is a daily form of self-love and respect that negates anxiety.

Additional tools of discovery:

1. Practice saying "No" three times a week for a month. Part of saying no is getting over the fear that the world will end or that people will hate you. So, practice with

strangers first and then work your way up to your loved ones.

2. Affirmations. Use these words or create your own. Use daily.

"I am trusting myself to have my back more each day."

"I honor needs in myself and others."

"I am enjoying my self-care more every day."

CHAPTER 7

Sovereignty

"Nothing binds you except your thoughts; nothing limits you
except fear; and nothing controls you except your beliefs."
– Marianne Williamson

The Sovereignty of a Queen means self-authority, autonomy, and personal freedom. Anxiety cannot survive well in this territory at all. The next step to clearing our mind and attaining this autonomy is to have some supportive guidelines that can help us align our minds with our true values. We will do this in a few different ways.

The Freedom of the Four Agreements

First, we will concentrate on the Toltec traditions of *The Four Agreements* by Don Miguel Ruiz, who I took the opportunity to closely study with for eight years in the mid-eighties(1). These agreements are a wonderful framework to clarify and strengthen our mental capacity. They encourage us become more aware in our Witness and stop our ego's unconscious thoughts and behaviors. We are here to be our best Self, and we cannot be that if we are suffering from our mind's beliefs and thoughts.

Practice #1: Cultivating Personal Authority

1. *Be impeccable with your word.* This means being true, honest, and centered with yourself. You don't say "Yes" when you mean "No." You use your boundaries and speak your truth the best you can. It also means you don't use words to go against yourself or others, as in gossiping and judging. Be aware that words have energy and power. Purposely align your words with your higher consciousness and love.

2. *Don't take things personally.* Recognize that people unknowingly project onto each other from our own inner stories and struggles. What people do or say isn't about you. It is about themselves and their lives. Stop hurting yourself. Use your mental boundaries to stop getting caught up in people's stories. Choose to focus on yourself, your thinking, and your behavior instead.

3. *Don't make assumptions.* Ask questions and clarify before you respond in situations. Be present and get out of your head. Avoid the drama that happens when we make assumptions and decisions without having all of the information. Have respect for yourself and others to communicate as clearly and as honestly as you can.

4. *Always do your best.* This means showing up every day to do the best you can with your level of health, energy, and consciousness on that day. Don't feel sorry for yourself or give yourself room to play a victim. Keep growing and learning. As we evolve, we live with more awareness, capacity, and alignment with our True Self.

These agreements take time to internalize. Our ego mind will resist them. The key is persistence and self-devotion. How much do you want to stop suffering? These agreements have the capability to provide us with incredible energy, support, and freedom from anxiety if we choose to apply them. They help us execute our authority with ourselves and our minds. They foster our Queen sensibilities and self-honor that comes with sovereignty.

Unknowingly, Jacqueline, age 32, was very caught up in gossip as part of her family culture. She expresses how annoyed she gets with her family but couldn't name why. As she studies the Four Agreements, she is realizing that it is the gossiping, judgments, and assumptions which are commonplace in her family that drive her crazy. She is figuring out how she can stay out of it, take care of herself, and not make her family wrong. It is taking time, and she is finding that she can be around them in small doses and keep practicing maintaining her boundaries and energy. This is a feat! And the good news is our personal changes often ripple out and begin to influence others around us, unconsciously.

The Power of Your Belief System

Another way we support our self-authority is when we can act like the hostess of our mind and consider our personalities and beliefs as guests. Without supervision and boundaries, the ego and the IC can get tyrannical. They are like two-year-olds who think they're the boss of the place. When we forget whose mind it is, we lose control of the throne in a big way. There is nothing worse than feeling that we are a slave of our own mind. This happens when we are not in charge of what we are putting our attention on. We must reclaim our authority. It doesn't mean we need to go to war and imprison these parts. It just means we need to learn to act smarter, and nicely put them into places of less power.

We begin by naming our mind's parts. The beauty of discovering more about these parts is that they, of course, are us. And the more we know about ourselves, the more we can care for ourselves. We also want to notice what areas of our body get activated when different beliefs are running us. For example, when my perfectionist part shows up, I usually feel a tightness in my neck and stomach. Then I know she is present and I need to talk with her. If I feel her approaching, then I can be proactive. This of course, benefits us with our anxiety. The more we know about our mind and body, the better we can address what we need to do to stay in charge.

Practice #2: Addressing Your Primary Beliefs

Training in observing your belief systems, happens from your Witness awareness. This allows you to see what is actually happening, which you can't do if you are in denial or stuck in a reaction pattern with those parts. It is best to do when you are calm at first. You start by taking inventory of your beliefs and fear stories, and name them so you can identify them clearly and succinctly.

Take out a sheet of paper and draw a vertical line down the middle. Identify your most noticeable belief systems that are creating problems for you: i.e., Fearful Frida, or Anxious Annie, or Critical Cathy. Use your awareness to determine the most important ones to focus on currently. For example, my perfectionist part that makes me crazy, I call Perfectionistic Patty. She believes that for me to be OK and safe in the world I must be perfect. When I was a kid, she was part of my coping strategy to deal with the chaos around me. I would put this description about her in the left column. I also would add how she thinks and how my body is affected by her thinking.

Add a few more primary negative beliefs in the left column. Write in the qualities of each personality to the best of your ability. Under each belief, write a description of the primary thinking patterns associated with it. Add to it as you identify more characteristics of that belief. Fill out all five negative beliefs first, then go back and find the perfect name like Fred, Jack, or Julie that works for you. Naming them keeps it light-hearted and makes it easier to identify them, as we face these treacherous old belief patterns. We can relate to them as parts of us.

A fun way to work with the parts is to have an active dialogue with them. One method is to dialogue with the parts from locations of your body parts where they resonate the most. For example, I can dialogue with Patty the Perfectionist, whose voice I would say relates with my neck, and speak with my Compassionate Cindy who I feel lives in my heart chakra. I go back and forth as if this is two people are negotiating a new agreement. Another format to dialogue with is journaling the conversation with writing and taking turns speaking for each part by feeling their position, not just thinking it.

As you become more conscious of your primary beliefs, you can transform them or you can learn to let go of the ones that no longer serve you. After practicing a while, you will begin to feel your authority returning. Then you will be able to catch what is happening in your internal dialogue instead of it unconsciously running you. For example, when my Perfectionistic Patty is sneaking up and starting with the, "You really should do that better because it doesn't look good enough…" I can respond with, "Patty, I hear you, but I don't worry about that stuff anymore. I really prefer you to tell me that it's good enough for now, and let me focus on what is more important." This invites the positive version for Patty to say to me, "That is good enough, Kate." I can let her down easy, instead of attacking her and saying "Go away you witch!" If you resist it, it will persist. Patty will persist in the negative light if I just try to ignore her. If I cajole her into seeing how her role could be more effective in a slightly different way, she will not feel as threatened. You learn to not engage the negative belief pattern and instead give your attention to the positive aspects. The negative belief core pattern will lose its power over time.

Wanda, a 31-year-old hard-working single mother of a six-year-old daughter, struggles with horrible self-esteem and anxiety issues. She is addressing her martyr belief that feeling sorry for herself is a helpful coping strategy. She was raised by a mom who was a very miserable martyr, so she feels unable to shake it off as her default belief. Whenever things get challenging, she gets lost in this wave of self-pity that spirals her down. As Wanda trains in noticing this pattern, she is getting much better at catching it. She is recently noticing how Maggie, the Martyr, is not around as much. She is shocked how it is working. I said "You are putting in the time and effort and it makes a difference."

Practice #3: Re-Assign Your Advisory Committee

As a Queen, it is time to elect the beliefs you want and need the most on your primary advisory committee. Which ones do you trust, and which are going to be the most helpful to you right now in your life? Whichever ones are not helpful should be demoted and given clear limits.

You also want to start identifying new beliefs that you may be lacking in your psyche. Look at what is missing in your life. Is it nurturing? Is it a loving, masculine aspect? Create some new personalities like Nurturing Nancy or Sweet Sam as voices that you want to have on your new committee to support you in your new way of life.

Julie, a 42-year-old successful entrepreneur, loves making up names for her beliefs. She enjoys creating new aspects of her old beliefs to support her better with her anxiety. She has developed Calming Connie and Soothing Steven to be her new advocates on her committee. She told me how the more she connects with these new aspects, the more powerful they are able to assist her when she is struggling to reset herself.

As we develop the advisory committee that strengthens and encourages us, this keeps us in charge and aware our needs. Once you have regained the throne of your Mind, it will eventually reflect in your external reality as well. Your self-image and your relationships to people, work, and life will demonstrate this inner conviction and self-authority. Now we get to move to the Body dimension next, the territory of the Heroine principle.

Main Messages:

1. Sovereignty requires the Queen to rule her belief systems.
2. With practice, we can stop feeding the negative beliefs and reinforce supportive ones.
3. The Queen must designate her trustworthy, loyal advisory committee.

Additional Tools of Discovery:

1. Draw a hierarchy or mind map of your primary belief systems with you as the Queen. Put it in a way that makes sense to you, so that you decide who has more or less power and who gets to show up and when. Or, have a meeting out loud in your living room with your advisory committee and figure out the new boundaries.
2. Affirmations. Try these or use your own wording:
   "As Queen, I am in charge of myself and my mind."
   "I am making good decisions for myself every day."
   "I am loving myself when I set my boundaries."

PART THREE

The Heroine

"There are always these moments in life when the limits of suffering are reached and we become heroes and heroines."

– Katherine Mansfield

CHAPTER 8

The Body Dimension

"The eagle has no fear of adversity. We need to be like the eagle
and have a fearless spirit of a conqueror!"

– Joyce Meyer

The Heroine principle is the aspect of our inner spiritual warrior self. She is the part of us that is tired of suffering and is willing to do what it takes to make it better. She is the fearless part of us that has been oppressed, repressed, and suppressed over thousands of years of the patriarchy. She is necessary to our wholeness and freedom. It is time to reclaim the essence of our feminine power inside of us and our bodies. Most Goddess-based cultures, before the patriarchal times, lived with gender equality and harmony among men and women with values of respect for each other, nature, the Earth, the elements and life(1). The feminine principle was honored by everyone. Hopefully, this is where we are heading again.

The Heroine archetype is the part of us who remembers when the fall of feminine power and respect happened thousands of years ago. The split within men from their own feminine sides and the deep oppression of women that has led to our world being significantly out of balance in its values, morals, and ethics. Today, people are more dissociated from their bodies, nature, and Mother Earth than ever before. We attain our sense of identity from our financial or marital status, our homes, and cars. The body has become an object to judge, manipulate, and disregard. Feminine values of creativity, connection, relationship, intuition, and embodiment have been marginalized and dismissed as weak and futile.

However, in the last ten years, scientific research has been validating the superior function of these feminine traits of intuition and mindfulness for accessing new ideas and creative problem solving methods, that are making businesses think twice(2). In addition, it has been shown that mind-body self-care is instrumental in reducing stress and healthcare costs as well as increasing work productivity(3). In other words, feminine qualities are now being scientifically recognized as valuable to the corporate world and mainstream culture. We may have a chance of changing as a society back to a healthy balance of masculine and feminine principles and values.

How does this fit in with anxiety? The dissociation, disconnection, and disembodiment that have resulted from our unhealthy culture are all related to people's anxiety. Dissociation teaches us that when we are feeling uncomfortable, we should go take a pill, have a drink, get high, binge on Netflix, go shopping.... We are taught young to become consumers who want and need the next thing to feel OK. We are told that people cannot tolerate feeling upset and need medication. This is a dangerous story that has led us to today's modern people who cannot deal with life not going their way. In reality, we are fully capable of feeling distress and coping with it and recovering ourselves. But many of us have forgotten how.

Disconnection also relates to the loss of our own internal values and what is important to us. Our culture's mainstream message is that we need to belong and conform more than stand out, be different, or hold onto our uniqueness. This leads to us giving up our own values and taking on the ones around us, just to fit in. Then we are disconnected from who we are and what we actually need. This leads to many problems including anxiety and depression, which is rampant worldwide.

Disembodiment speaks to the ways we cut off our connection to our own bodies, the Earth, and our sense of self. Our culture has such a distorted obsession with money and power that the elemental joys and beauty of simply being are minimized and forgotten. The pleasures of shared time with people we love are obscured with ever-present technology. The ways we can be nurtured in nature are no longer valued. We become disembodied in ourselves, within our communities, and as human beings.

This Heroine principle is our hidden cry for help to reclaim ourselves, our bodies, and a way of life that supports us. She is our savior, here to teach us how we can be embodied once again and revere our bodies as sacred ground.

Part Three explores Reverence for our bodies as we learn about our own anxiety sensation patterns. We then focus on the Wisdom of our emotional intelligence and how feelings need to be sensed in our bodies to adequately address our anxiety. In the last section of the Heroine, we delve into the element of Courage as the force that carries us through our fears to the other side in a loving and powerful way.

CHAPTER 9

───

Reverence

"The body is precious. It is our vehicle for awakening. Treat it with care."
– Buddha

Our bodies are our uncharted and greatest allies. They deserve to be held in reverence. The Heroine archetype cannot fully express herself without us being fully aligned with our bodies. In other words, our bodies are necessary for reaching our fullest power and potential as a Heroine.

In our culture, we generally do not treat our bodies reverently. Our bodies endure a lot from us. The get pushed around, ignored, undernourished, judged, unappreciated, abused, and disrespected. Most of us are bullies and blame our bodies. With our anxiety, it is no different. We shame our bodies for being weak and powerless in the face of anxiety. We get mad at it for shaking and freaking out. We make it the body's fault we feel this way, when really, our bodies are incredibly loyal to us. What if we were as loyal to our bodies in return? How come we aren't?

We grew up this way. We saw our family treat their bodies this way. We live in a culture that is all about regarding the body as an object, which contributes to our society's highest levels ever of chronic health issues, pain, and illness. We are taught to feel ashamed for having a body that doesn't reflect Hollywood perfection. It is an object that is just supposed to be useful to us. It's not a part of us. It is like a purse, an accessory, that we are required to take with us everywhere. We completely miss the natural wisdom and consciousness of the body, and its real purpose.

Our body takes on the suffering of anxiety because that's all it can do, until we wake up and pay attention to why it is happening. Our bodies do not initiate anxiety; they are simply responding to the directive of the mind to be prepared for danger, whether it is real or not. First let's look at how to appreciate our bodies.

Nourishing Your Body-Love

The truth is that the body is our sacred ground. It is the home for our Heroine, our soul, our heart, and our mind in this lifetime. We each only have one body and we can't trade it in and buy a new one. It is truly devoted to us, unlike our ego, which is quite undependable and turns on us regularly. Our body carries all our memories in its cells. It is our blueprint of life, and it can be our map for healing as well. However, we need to decide if we are willing to stop treating as a shameful servant, like Dobby in the Harry Potter books. Our bodies cannot be our sacred ground, powerful and healing, until we learn how to care and show up for it. When we stop the shaming and blaming of our body and give it some respect and say, "I am going to try to love you and be more kind to you," our bodies immediately respond with, "I have been waiting all my life to hear you say that!" This is like the secret pathway that won't open without the magic words. These are the magic words: "I love you and I will care for you." Once we say this, our body in all its infinite wisdom is our champion. It will do what it takes to help us get out of our suffering. It is full of resources and experiences that can connect us with who we truly are. Our bodies are also our secret weapon in freeing ourselves from of our anxiety.

Self-care from the body perspective is necessary, especially for women trying to reduce their anxiety. The importance of entering a state of physical relaxation as well as psychologically disconnecting from daily stressors has been found to be an essential component of our wellbeing(1). Most of us do not even give ourselves time to get to all our errands, forget downtime, right? This is the thinking that needs to change. We looked at self-care from the mental perspective in the prior chapters. Let's briefly talk about body self-care as it relates with anxiety. Physical self-care includes how we move, how we breathe, how we eat, how we sleep, and how we are present and grounded in our bodies. It also relates to how we make physical contact and get touched, hugged, and are sexually involved. It is associated with our time in nature and off technology screens. When we are struggling with anxiety, we need to be aware of choosing the healthiest and most loving options for ourselves. This is what is necessary, not indulgent, if you are wanting to diminish anxiety.

Sam, a 43-year-old high achieving executive came to me about her anxiety and her inability to sleep well. As we explore her sleep issues, we are identifying a few surprising patterns. When Sam does not take quiet time away from work and her computer in the evening, her body cannot wind down enough to fall asleep. And if she is sexual with someone she does not care for, she will get agitated and restless afterwards and cannot sleep through the night. As she is addressing these behaviors and experimenting with new habits, her sleep is improving and her anxiety is lessening. Sam sees now that her body was trying to communicate with her all along and she didn't know how to listen.

The more aware we are of our bodies and what they need, the more powerful of an ally our bodies can be for us. Our bodies are the container for our mental, emotional, and spiritual well-being. How we treat our bodies, reflects directly with whether we are cherishing it or diminishing it. Let's see about how the body communicates with us through the language of sensations.

The Language of Sensations

Training our mind to notice and pay attention to the sensations of our bodies is important and can take practice. For some of us who have been dissociated from our bodies for most of our lives, we may feel more numbness and frozenness in our bodies. Start with that sensation. At first, we may observe when we feel hot or cold and temperature variations. Then move onto identifying tension and tightness in the body. Eventually, our awareness and vocabulary will expand as we get to know our body's language of sensations.

Practice #1: Name the Sensations of Anxiety

First, let's recognize how anxiety feels in your body. Think of the last experience you had with anxiety as if it were happening now. How does it show up in your body? As sweaty palms, racing heart, or tense hands in the beginning? Does it lead to blurred vision, feeling disoriented, and difficulty breathing? Just pay attention and write down a list.

See if you can organize the sensations into the early, middle, and late phases of your anxiety symptoms. Now see what your mind is usually saying to you when you are having these sensations; maybe "the world is over" or "I'm dying" or something else like that. When the mind makes up these catastrophic stories, the body will respond accordingly with, "Oh no, let's run from the danger!" The body is not invested in you being terrified. It doesn't like to have to run to stay safe. But some of us blame the body as the culprit for our anxiety. We punish it like it is the body's fault for making us feel stressed, uncomfortable, and frightened. Remember those pesky beliefs we named in the Mind section: They are the culprits.

Our bodies' sensations are literally our warning signals that something is happening inside of us and we are not detecting the mind's beliefs that are triggering the physical responses. Many people do not sense their warning signs. They are not present enough in their bodies to catch the early stages of anxiety. Being dissociated eventually will lead to anxiety, so it becomes a catch-22 cycle. The mind gets triggered with fear, then the physiological response of fight or flight happens in the body, and then the mind escalates further. When we develop our body awareness, anxiety becomes an alarm to alert us that we need to pay attention and see if it is a belief, a feeling a sensation, a memory, a need etc. This how we can use anxiety to our advantage.

My dear client Susan has horrible panic and anxiety attacks. She never knows where they are coming from. She gets sideswiped by anxiety and feels frozen in her tracks. She shakes, her heart rate increases, and her palms start sweating with panic running through her. She dislikes her body and does not value her body. It is just another thing to take care of. It feels like a burden. In her sessions, we focus on her connecting with her body in new ways. As she is using her grounding and embodiment practices, Susan is reporting that she is starting to feel calmer. The more consistent she practices and feels her body, the more she is appreciating all it does for her. Now she can work with the emotional aspects of her anxiety. When I saw her recently, she looked like a different person. She is carrying herself in a completely new way. She said she is seeing how her anxiety is a warning signal that she has become spaced out and ungrounded. She feels more confident she can do something to change it now.

The Gift of Body Presence

Embodiment practices are a fundamental part of most wisdom school traditions. They are considered an integral process of healing, wholeness, and spiritual development for human beings. New research shows us how grounding and Earthing are powerful embodiment skills that are incredibly helpful for our wellbeing, physical health, mental states, and moods(2,3). Earthing is the grounding we do by being in physical in contact with the Earth's surface. Researchers note that Earthing creates an electrical conductive response that directly relates to changes in mood, inflammation, immune responses, wound healing, and treatment of autoimmune diseases(4,5). In this Fear-Less approach, embodiment is key to accessing our Heroine and healing the physical and emotional aspects of ourselves.

Practice #2: Embodiment as a Daily Practice

Grounding means becoming present in your body. To practice grounding, pick a time when you can focus on being present and not be interrupted. You can start by becoming aware of your breath moving in and out of your body. Relax your muscles. Focus on your feet. Imagine you are sending down roots like a tree, deep into the Earth.

Then bring your attention to the sensations in the rest of your body. Begin noticing areas of tension, and allow your breath to help it flow down through your feet and out into the Earth below. It is the awareness that matters here. Your thinking becomes clearer, your presence deeper, and your energy more accessible. You can ground by doing a body scan, by running, by stretching, by dancing, by making love. It is focusing your attention on your body's experience that makes it magical. Grounding directly impacts anxiety in a positive way. Practicing grounding means you can begin being more present and conscious in your body, with more of your resources available.

I think of it as being a whole-person instead of being a bodiless head walking around.

Earthing, on the other hand, means to be at a place on the Earth's surface where you can contact the ground directly on dirt, sand, or rock, without shoes. Repeat the above instructions for grounding practice. Be aware of the energetic experience from the direct contact with the planet. Notice any energy shifts inside you, on your skin, or in your auric field. Be mindful. Thank Mother Earth. Thank your body. They are the same.

My client Sue has anxiety from recently losing her husband of 50 years. She has a hard time being in her body due to past childhood trauma. When I suggest she find a tree in the park near her house where she can sit and get grounded and release some grief, she looks at me like I am crazy. I just say, "It's up to you if you want to try it." A few weeks later, she casually mentions that she did find a good tree. I ask her how it is. She says it is good. I don't push it. I am just glad she is open to trying it. Now it is a regular part of how she grounds and feels less overwhelmed when she is missing her husband. I am grateful she can get some relief with Mother Earth.

The Efficacy of the Breath

Our breath is another vital way we get embodied. Physiologically, our breath enables us to actively shift our nervous system's responses to life experiences. Our central nervous system is either in Sympathetic (SNS), which is active and alert, or Parasympathetic (PNS), which is the relaxation response. In Kundalini Yoga, the system of Pranayama, or breath-work, makes up one of the eight limbs of Yoga. Breath-work can directly impact our brains, bodies, moods, and our ability to regulate our emotions(6). It has been scientifically validated as a very powerful tool for people with anxiety(7,8). Breathwork impacts anxiety by deactivating the SNS that gets stuck in overdrive, feeding us adrenaline like we are running from a bear. Focused breathing stimulates the relaxation response of the PNS, allowing our heart rate and blood pressure to lower and our fight or flight symptoms to calm down. Below, I show you the foundational breathing techniques that help anxiety.

Practice #3: Engaging Your Relaxation Response

a) Full Breath Breathing. First, let's practice deep breathing into the three sections of the lungs that allow more air and life force (prana) into our bodies. When we breathe shallowly, we do not take in enough prana, which leads to us being tired more often. We drink caffeine to get "energy" and it drains the adrenals, shortens the breath even more, and leads to a bigger energy crash.

To begin this practice, find a place to lay down that is quiet and undisturbed. If you are not new to this, stay sitting up with a straight spine. Put your hands on your lower belly, below the navel. First, breathe into the area between your collar bones and your chest. Do this 3-5 times. Then, breathe into the ribs and the diaphragm area. Do this 3-5 times. Then try focusing your breathing into the lower lungs, so that the lower belly fills up and rises as you inhale and falls back down as you exhale. Do this 3-5 times. Do not pressure yourself. Relax and do your best, it's good enough. Then try breathing with all three areas of the lungs. Fill the top of the lungs first, then the mid-section and then the lower belly. Then release from the lower belly first, and as the belly recedes towards the spine, then relax the ribs, and then lower the collarbone as you exhale out the top of the lungs. This takes some practice, but can be a good meditation for relaxation, as well as before going to sleep at night or in the morning before you rise.

The impact of learning to breathe this way will grow every time you work with it. It can slow the mind, relax the body, reduce anxiety, and open creativity. Once you master the Full Breath breathing you can try Complete Breath breathing, sitting up with a straight spine. This breath begins by filling the lower lungs and belly first, then the mid lungs and fills up to the top of the collarbones last. When you release you slowly start at the top of the lungs, then release the air in the mid lungs and lastly in the low lungs as the belly recedes. Notice how your body responds differently.

b) Left Nostril Breathing: Sit with your spine straight and body relaxed. Keep your chin slightly tucked so that your neck aligns with your spine. Feel your sits bones under your buttocks connected with the Earth beneath you. Gently hold your right index finger or thumb and close off your right nostril. Begin breathing in slow, long, and deep through the left nostril. Then exhale out the left nostril in the same slow, long, and deep breath. Continue this breath for 3 minutes minimum for beneficial effect. Attend to the sensations or count the pace of the breath to keep your mind focused. This breath activates the relaxation response and slows you down. This breath is helpful for sleep disturbances, overwhelm, and sped-up thinking(8,9).

Naomi, age 57, is an extraordinary artist I met. She is going through menopause, gets bad hot flashes, anxiety, and heart palpitations, and she wants relief without medication and its side effects. I suggested some yogic breathing techniques, especially the Victory breath (described below). She is clearly motivated to stop suffering, so we practice it in each session. She expresses some relief right away. I told her that the more she practices, the more powerful an effect she will have. The next time I saw her, she had practiced in 3-4 times a day for two weeks straight. She says it is miraculous because she can start the victory breath as soon as she feels a hot flash coming and her body will relax and can bypass it. Her anxiety continues to reduce and she rarely has heart palpitations any more. I was so glad she was open to something out of her usual experience.

Our Heroine rules the domain of the Body, and she reveals the essential ways to be connected. As we become more aware of our body and its amazing capacity to support us and guide us through anxiety and life's challenges, we can increase our ability to love and accept it for the sacred vessel it is. Next, we will explore the essential language of feelings and sensations in the body as our next skill to serve us.

Main Messages:

1. The Heroine shows us that our body is our greatest ally.
2. When we revere our bodies, anxiety can be our early warning system.
3. Practicing embodiment and breath-work daily is essential for self-care.

Additional Tools of Discovery:

1. The Victory Breath. This breath is a part of an anxiety Kundalini yoga protocol that has been researched and verified. It can be easily done anywhere because you can do it with your eyes open. You start by breathing in a ¾ breath and holding it gently while you internally vibrate the word "victory" in three syllables: VIC-TOR-RY. Then exhale and repeat. Continue this breath for a minimum of three minutes or until you get the desired effect. This allows the fearful and compulsive thinking patterns to subside and the body to release tension(7).

2. Affirmations. Try these or use your own wording.

   "I am learning to listen to and love my body."

   "I am accepting and appreciating my body more every day."

   "My body is my ally in healing my anxiety."

CHAPTER 10

Wisdom

"Our inner guidance comes to us through our feelings and the body first, not through intellectual understanding."
– Christiane Northrup

Our Heroine represents our embodied wise woman part of us as well. She helps us take the necessary action to us where we want to go. She operates through the body and our emotions. This may be new territory for many of us, and she will show you the way.

How we grow up in our family environment teaches us how to relate to ourselves and others. Most of us, unfortunately, come from families where feelings were not validated or tolerated, let alone supported to be expressed freely. This is a result of our parents growing up in the same environment, or worse. The idea of knowing what you are feeling and why, which is now called Emotional intelligence (EQ), was not even a concept until the last 20 years.

Emotions are the lost language of our Heroine. Decades of research have now shown that EQ is not only essential for healthy personal development, but can also be a predictor of our mental health and professional efficacy(1,2). Emotional intelligence impacts how we take care of ourselves, manage our behaviors, navigate through social situations, and make personal decisions about what is best for us. It's important to know our feelings and how they inform us. Yet most of us didn't learn it. It's OK, we can develop it now, dear Heroine.

Befriending Your Feelings

Knowing when we are experiencing feelings and then discerning which feelings they are is a valuable skill for everyone, but especially folks with anxiety. Why? Because when people with anxiety cannot separate out and identify their different feelings, it becomes a huge yarn ball of emotions and sensations that habitually is associated with anxiety. We often have no idea what we are feeling or why we are feeling it when anxiety hits. By the time we notice anxiety is upon us, it kicks into gear with the physical symptoms that lead us back into old fears, and the cycle continues. When we can't track what we are feeling or what's going on, it is pretty easy for our fear stories to take us over. We decide we don't know what is happening and therefore have no power over it. This is what leads to chronic anxiety.

"Feelings Are Bad News" Myths

It's true that our culture dislikes feelings in general. We don't know how to relate to them, and we don't like receiving feelings from others, mostly because we don't feel adept at it. It is a social, cultural, and interpersonal dilemma that leads to anxiety.

There is a feelings myth in this culture that if we feel and express our feelings directly, we are going to hurt others, so we shouldn't do it. It will just make us feel like we are bad, guilty people. Let me ask you, are you more kind to people by being dishonest and unclear? Not really. Are these important relationships that matter to you, and do you want them to be trustworthy? How can there be actual trust if these people don't know what is going on for you? Failing to disclose your truth will end badly for any situation eventually, and will only lead to more anxiety for you.

Another idea people have is that if we can just ignore our bad feelings, they will go away. We don't want to feel our feelings because our ego tells us it will just make us more anxious. Then we get into the habit of deflecting, avoiding, and repressing our feelings, which unfortunately is part of what has gotten us into this cycle of anxiety in the first place. Feelings never go away if they have not been acknowledged, felt, and released. If we ignore them, they are not processed through. Instead, they are stored in the body. This is especially true for what we call shadow feelings, like anger, hurt, sadness, and fear.

Our shadow feelings are not bad. They are just the ones that society says are not OK because we don't know how to relate to them in a positive way. We avoid feeling them, even though they are perfectly normal, healthy feelings to have. When we ignore them, they will still demand our attention and come out some other way. This is part of the process behind how our anxiety grows huge and takes over. Feelings we don't know how to deal with get suppressed, avoided, and ignored. Then they come out as fears and sensations that we still are uncomfortable with – but they help us keep avoiding the real feelings underneath that we don't want to face. These disregarded feelings will slowly or not so slowly begin to manifest in the mind-body as some kind of dis-ease, discontent, or illness. This has become the status quo in our culture: to avoid and pay the price later, then be shocked when we are in pain and sick.

Handling feelings differently is a choice. We can either keep being afraid of our true feelings and face the consequences, or become empowered and able to respond to our feelings in a way that supports us. The process is the same as we have covered in other chapters: To acknowledge what is happening, allow it to unfold and awaken to the bigger picture of what we are genuinely needing.

Growing Your Emotional Intelligence

Emotional intelligence(EQ) means learning about our feelings and seeing them as the key to our ability to take care of ourselves and manage our life. When we have EQ, we become more socially aware and able to read people, to be a good judge of character, and to be empathic(1). We can take things less personally and are less easily offended. We can also say "no" and have boundaries. We can let go of our own mistakes rather than dwelling on them, as well as not holding grudges against others' mistakes. We know these qualities greatly assist people with anxiety.

High-EQ folks have learned to release perfection as a goal and be more accepting of themselves and others. These strategies help them keep their negative self-talk in check and stay in touch with their self-worth and joy. As a result, high-EQ people have improved interpersonal relations and greater life satisfaction(2,3). Emotional intelligence in the Fear-Less program needs to be related to the body to be most effective.

Practice #1: Naming Feelings and Related Bodily Sensations

Our first practice is identifying feelings and sensations in your own unique way. There is no right way. Sit and breathe and center in your body. Connect with your Witness mind. Take a moment and decide what your intent is for getting to know your feelings and what you would like to receive from the experience. Connect with your body and breathe from a place of appreciation. Give yourself permission to be uncomfortable. Start scanning your body for sensations or emotions. Keep coming back to your Witness awareness, naming and ignoring the chatty mind. You are not trying to control, stop, or avoid feelings. Your focus is to acknowledge the feelings and then allow them to express and flow through you. You may or may not know what they are related to. That is perfectly fine.

Start with a positive emotion i.e., "I feel satisfied with that meal," for instance. What does that feel like in your body? Take a few minutes and notice sensations that feel related to "I am satisfied in this moment." Experience it physically, emotionally, even energetically. As you practice this awareness it will become easier to see and name sensations as hot, tingly, numb, tense, nauseous, pointy, etc.

On a piece of paper, write down three to five feelings that you're feeling and their descriptive names. For each feeling, describe the physical sensations and experience of each feeling. See if you can determine the places in your body that you tend to associate with that feeling, i.e., I feel joy in my belly as cool, tingly energy. Do this for each feeling. You might recall a memory of when you felt it. You can envision it and recapture the full experience of that feeling so you can record details. Once you're complete with your exploration of that feeling, thank it for showing you more about yourself. Invite the next feeling in your body consciousness. When you are done, close this process with gratitude for yourself and your willingness to be curious and open.

Facing our shadow feelings can be more difficult at first. Learning how to be present with our grief, our fears, our rage, and our hurt is a human skill we desperately need to be proficient at to live as empowered women. Try out the above directions with a small shadow feeling first. Walk through the same steps and write it down. Thank it and yourself.

Joan, who is 69, is a bright, intellectual woman. She has had to dampen her emotions to survive her family as a child. Now she struggles with feeling numb and disconnected emotionally and physically. We practice these methods slowly to build her awareness and safety, so that she can gently release the numbing protection armor that she has worn all her life. She let me know she can feel tiny sensations in her body more and her heart is feeling a little more open and warm. This is no small deed for someone who has lived her whole life anesthetized. She can feel her painful feelings now without being embarrassed and ashamed. Her Heroine will get her there slowly but surely.

Practice #2: Creating Your Personal Feelings Range (0-10)

When you can recognize and know your range of a certain emotion, like fear, for example, it becomes your basis to identify what level of fear you are at on a scale from 0-10, with ten being the most fear and zero being none at all. This gives you essential information and a way to strategize. When you know you are at a 2 of fear that you call "concerned" versus being at a 6 which for you call "terrified," this gives you incredible power to act on what you need. You can improve your self-care dramatically with this tool.

***NOTE: If this feels too challenging to do alone, don't worry. I recommend having the support of a professional initially. Processing trauma is so important and needs to be done in a safe, secure environment with a professional you can trust.*

Start with centering in your body. Stay connected and conscious with your breath. Set your intent about what you want to get out of this practice. Pick the easiest shadow feeling you have, the one that's least triggering. On a piece of paper, draw a scale from zero to ten. Decide on words to call the zero and 10 of your scale. Don't overthink it, you can always update them later when you can have a thesaurus handy. Stay present in the moment. Put yourself inside of a memory when you had that feeling recently, so you're not just in your head about it.

Notice the sensations in your body. Then, find your 5 and add in what comes easily.

Try it out and think of a recent situation when you felt this feeling. Recognize how you moved up or down the scale of that emotion over a period of time. How could you become more aware and take pauses on that scale? How could that help you from becoming unconscious and lost in that feeling? Which strategies of grounding, stopping the fear stories, or setting boundaries could help you stay on the lower end of that scale, where you can have more control?

Emotional Body Pain

When we don't know how to process feelings, they can show up in the body as pain. In his book *The Mind-Body Prescription*, Dr. John Sarno wrote about this experience of the body-mind connection he saw repeatedly in his practice in the early 1970s(4). People came to Dr. Sarno with back, neck, or leg pain that was usually chronic. What he noticed was that most everyone of these people had one thing in common: They had repressed emotions, usually anger. As he included counseling in his program with patients, he saw people have dramatic changes in their pain levels or complete remission of symptoms. He hypothesized that people who couldn't cope with their emotions unconsciously allowed the mind to relocate the emotions into the body as pain in an attempt to distract from those emotions. He told patients who were open to the idea that they could choose to stay in physical pain, or they could acknowledge and face the emotional pain and see it through.

He saw amazing results where people's chronic pain could be gone in a few sessions.

Teri, a 39-year-old woman with fibromyalgia, works with me on this very issue. She initially was very reticent to hear about repressed feelings being related to body pain. This concept made her angry, as she felt it blamed her for getting herself sick. We worked through this many times; that she is not to blame, but she is responsible for her mind, body, and spirit. She knows she has my greatest compassion. It is not an easy situation to face. The more she is willing to experiment with identifying feelings and expressing them in a safe, clear way, the more she feels her physical symptoms change. It doesn't mean that her fibromyalgia will all go away, but it doesn't mean that it couldn't, either. It is a personal relationship for each of us to unravel and decide what we want to believe and what we are willing to let go of.

Recent research has verified this same view of Dr. Sarno, with chronic low back pain being highly associated with poor emotional processing skills of suppressed fear, anxiety, or anger(5). Chronic pain is the messenger of many complex, suppressed emotions that need nurturing, safe places to be heard(6). When we choose to be responsible for our emotions, even if they are difficult and painful, we step into authority of our wellbeing. We can master strategies that will make us more conscious of our triggers, habits, and perceptions that do and do not serve us. First, we need to build up our tolerance for feeling our feelings.

Now that you have a scale for shadow feelings, let's practice feeling the different levels of that range. Learning to accept and bear our feelings is possible, when we do it slowly. Dr. Stephen Levine calls this "pendulating." In his book *Waking the Tiger*, he talks about the slow process of renegotiating our relationships with feelings and past trauma for the sake of clearing them from our bodies. Here, we are taking baby steps with acknowledging feelings and allowing them to be felt in small bits at a time. Gaining tolerance and aptitude for our emotions helps us learn more about ourselves, change unhealthy reactions and habits, and build new pathways in the brain that all serve to decrease our anxiety.

Practice #3: "Pendulating" with Your Emotion

Get quiet, centered, and aware of your Witness. Set your intention about learning how to be more tolerant of feelings your feelings. Now pick a negative feeling that is your easiest feeling you can relate to, not your hardest. Think of the most recent situation where you felt this feeling. Be aware to distance your ego, so you don't get caught in fear stories. Observe this memory from afar. You are not getting lost in it as if it is happening right now. It's more like watching a movie of the experience, with some distance. Stay present and focused on your breath, your body awareness, your sensations. Move towards it with curiosity and breathe. Be patient and open. Pay attention to any sensations. When the feeling begins to amplify, move back away from it. You are dipping your toe into the feeling and pulling it back out so you can soothe yourself. This is key. Learn to take care of yourself and grow your tolerance for facing this emotional content in a safe, slow way. Do this for five minutes at first. Then build up time with each practice session. Listen to your inner wisdom. Give yourself a hug and some appreciation for this important step.

With time, patience and practice, our emotional intelligence can develop and help us lessen our habitual anxiety responses. For now, fostering your ability to identify your feelings and their range is primary. The other work of EQ with empowering our boundaries and capacity for forgiveness comes later. Next, we delve into courage and compassion with our feelings as we develop our skills for healing and integration.

Main Messages

1. Our Heroine needs us to be fluent in our emotions so we can heal and be wise.

2. We develop our emotional intelligence by acknowledging feelings in our mind-body.

3. As we increase our EQ, we decrease our anxiety patterns.

Additional Tools of Discovery

1. Tapping. Tapping is an old technique for soothing the nervous system when it's activated with emotion and fear stories. Bilateral tapping is the best. It helps the mind-body process and regulate the experience. Tap with two hands at both sides under the collar bones alternating contact. Or you can tap bilaterally on the knees or thighs. Focus on your breathing pace instead of thinking. Relax the body. Accept the emotion and allow it to flow through you.

2. Affirmations. Try these words or use your own.

"I am growing my emotional intelligence daily with attention and love."

"I am facing and accepting my feelings more every day."

"I can take care of and release my feelings with love."

CHAPTER 11

———

Courage

"It's like when you learn to swim by swimming.
You learn courage by couraging."
– Mary Daly

As our Heroine encourages us to face our feelings and sensations, we improve our ability to connect with all aspects of ourselves. For sure, there are some parts we would prefer not to hang out with too much. These are usually from our past when we felt miserable and did not know how to cope with the pain, or we didn't have adequate support for dealing with what was happening. Anxiety, for many folks, is related to these hurt sides of us. These denied, repressed, and wounded parts of us, however, are key for us to integrate if we want to lessen our anxiety and feel whole and powerful again. Our Heroine guides us on how to get through this to the other side.

Wanting to Check Out

Naturally, we want to run as fast as possible the other way from these old painful places. We don't want to deal with them. We try to avoid this step by caving into our ego's denial and telling ourselves that maybe anxiety is not that bad. It's no big deal. Just ignore the elephant in the room, right? But we know that all these repressed feelings will stir up anxiety again at some point very soon. Remember, survival mode takes an exhausting amount of energy each day just to keep afloat, stay in denial, and keep up the self-defeating stories. We have no real choices in survival mode. We know we can't shut down the pain without shutting down our entire emotional range as well. No hurt or anger also means no joy or happiness. We also realize we can only last so long here in survival mode before it will catch up with us. The body and mind can live in fear for only so long before there is a breakdown emotionally, physically, or spiritually. This is when we can have car accidents, get fired, or get ill.

Let's peek at the ways we are taught in our culture to pretend we are not checking out of life when we are. We can choose medication, substances, shopping, gambling, or overworking among many others. Society says we can just take a pill and then we don't have to deal with anything. The problem is that your body, mind, and spirit still deal with the pain and the feelings, even if your ego won't. Whatever story we have about how terrifying it would be to face what is inside of us is more an exaggerated version from our childhood fears. I'm not saying that life isn't challenging and pain isn't painful. But if we stay in the dark and ignore our wounds, we lose our power of choice and consciousness and that just makes life even tougher.

Remember that your Body is this spiritual warrior, and it was made for this. The courage to be vulnerable is the only way through to heal and stop the anxiety cycle.

Jill is an astute active 74-year-old woman I have the pleasure of working with. She struggles with her lifelong anxiety and depression she has had since childhood. She never feels worthy of love due to early wounding from her mother. Despite a long marriage, a successful career, and grown adult children and grandchildren whom she loves, Jill is stuck in self-loathing. Guiding her in facing her wounds with courage and compassion has been an amazing journey. The more she cultivates compassion for herself and her self-loathing, the more she lets the light in and the more she releases her old patterns of being. It truly is possible if you are dedicated. How can do we do this? We start with collecting our loyalty and support team.

Gathering Your Resources

Whenever we are doing deep internal work, we want to establish our resources for ourselves. Resources are the people, places, and things that support us, both externally and internally. They may be in our present life or from our past. They can be alive or dead. We call on our external resources by communicating with those trustworthy folks about what kind of support we may need from them. We also create our internal support network with a self-care plan and collecting our mental, emotional, physical, and spiritual resources. We want to get good sleep, eat a good meal, and be loving and nurturing with ourselves before we do this work, so we can be calm, receptive and open.

Practice #1: Calling in Assistance for Courage Work

First you call on the Courage of your inner Heroine.

We also want you have a sacred circle of support for yourself that creates a safe, secure, and centered space. Those resources might be people or pets from your life that you will energetically request to be in your circle. They can also be spiritual or archetypal. Consider asking your own Higher Self to help in this query. You can call on any spiritual teachers, angels, guides, or goddesses that you resonate with. Call them to come be here with you for this time. Show them where you want them to be in your circle as they arrive. Each time you plan to do this work, you call this circle to create a safe, quiet, contained space. Do this with intention and sacred presence for yourself. This is Courage work.

This is the feminine work you didn't know that you have been waiting for. Permission to show up for yourself and receive support in a way that is healing, loving, and accepting without any agenda. Sometimes you can get caught up in the idea that if someone else would just love you enough, your pain would go away. Unfortunately, it doesn't work that way. Facing what you disown and reject is a personal job. We can have our teammates but we are the captain of the ship. The only way to heal is within yourself, with your own love, compassion, and acceptance. You can do this, Heroine.

Katherine, a strong business woman, is coaching with me and ready to face her deeper Courage work so she can stop her consistent panic attacks. She has avoided it long enough and although she is scared still, she also has cultivated enough self-devotion to keep going. When I talk about how we start with calling in support, she rolls her eyes and gives me an "Are you kidding me?" look. I just repeat the instructions. We do it together in the session to help her move past her embarrassment and judgment. As soon as she starts calling in her support, tears began streaming down her face, which surprised her. This is what we all deeply want and never give ourselves: being loved, supported and receiving it fully. She did an amazing piece of healing work that day. She still jokes with me about the circle of support, but I know she got it.

Building Your Self-Compassion

It is through compassion that we transform our wounds. Courage is our self-compassion in action. What this means is that when we muster the courage to face our shadow parts and love and accept them with compassion, we become more integrated and whole inside. Self-compassion is self-acceptance, forgiveness, and appreciation of ourselves all rolled up in one. In her book, *Self-Compassion*, Kristen Neff shares a self-compassion scale that she created to help us understand how to develop this crucial healing stance with ourselves. When we begin to have self-compassion, this improves our ability to self-regulate our emotions, feel more confident, be less self-judgmental and have decreased anxiety and depression(1). When we practice it faithfully, it becomes an effective way to lower burn-out and promotes maintenance of our self-care(2). Self-compassion assists us in accomplishing our inner work to make our outer life less troublesome.

"Painful feelings are by their very nature temporary ... as long as we don't prolong or amplify through resistance or avoidance. The only way out to eventually free ourselves from debilitating pain, therefore, is to be with it as it is. The only way out is through."

– Kristen Neff

One place we all need to practice compassion is with our inner child part of ourselves. This work is about being the caring parent figure for our younger parts that we have left behind in past challenging situations. Our inner child deserves a special type of treatment from us. It may take us a while to cultivate the presence, love, and awareness for this process, but it is worth sticking with. We all have an inner child. Some of us may have a good relationship already. Many of us learned to deny their existence because it means remembering difficult life experiences that are painful. No matter how old you are, this inner child, if left miserable and unsupervised, can make our life hell. This part can easily derail any positive changes we want. Each person's inner child has its own personality, but they usually all feel a sense of being neglected, abandoned, and rejected from us. There is reparation work to be done. Many folks with traumatic childhoods believe they are better off not engaging with this part of themselves. But it never pans out. Ultimately, your inner child will refuse to be ignored. Lucky for you, that allows you to heal instead of staying split off, anxious, and miserable. It is the only road to true redemption, dear Heroine.

Practice #2: Connect with Your Inner Child

This is a practice that requires patience. If you have no current relationship with your inner child and you are starting from scratch, you will need to build rapport and trust one step at a time. Close your eyes and imagine a certain age of your child self that is NOT the most intense part of your life, but one you can more easily relate to. Introduce yourself. Say why you are reaching out. Begin to share about yourself. Acknowledge that you may not have known that it was important to be connected to her. For now, you are just holding space and creating connection.

Do this regularly, and take a bit more time each visit. Build safety. Create connection. Add in imaginary contact, hugging, and holding. Remember, the psyche doesn't distinguish from real or imagined. Imagine putting her in a fun, safe place when you leave to work. Take time to be playful and do things she wants to do when you can. Become more attentive to how to make her feel safe. Slowly work with different ages when you were in different places of hardship. Your biggest job is to be present, drop the judgment, and keep her safe. And when she acts out and suddenly has more control than you do, stop. It is as if she took the car keys and was going to drive. Stop her and put her in the back in a child seat, buckle her in, and give her a snack. Get in the driver's seat as your adult self. You are in charge again. Be the nurturing parent. Notice what changes occur, when you can hold these two perspectives consciously.

Keep working with her until it feels natural. It can lead to amazing inner peace.

Courage Work

We are building a relationship with our internal aspects of ourselves that we have not had the capacity or the awareness to do before. It may feel silly and fake at first, which is normal. But if you follow through with this, in a matter of days you can feel shifts happen under the surface, deep inside your psyche and body. This is called Courage work for a reason. You show up, do the best you can, and it's good enough.

Note: External professional resources may be a helpful support at times in this work. I would not have come through all I did in my life on my own. So, whether it's a counselor for trauma, a shaman for soul retrieval, a mind-body coach, or an energy worker for body emotional release, find a qualified, experienced, personally-referred resource and then meet them before you do work with them.

Practice #3: The Coming Home Process

One of my favourite processes is called "Ho-opono-pono," an ancient Hawaiian modality of healing(3). It is so subtle and yet incredibly powerful. There are many applications of this modality. I use it with clients as they call home the parts of themselves that they have lost, rejected, or disowned. The version I use brings the Ho-opono-pono process into the body and makes it more a physical expression. I call it the Coming Home Process.

To start, you create a safe space that is undisturbed. Get centered and grounded in your body. Find your breath.

Connect with your Witness awareness. Set your intention on the desired outcome. Call in your resources. Choose to work with a little wound, like an upset with a friend. Not the biggest, scariest one. Bring the incident to mind. Notice what feelings are present around this wound. It can be hurt, anger, fear, or sadness. Bring it to your awareness in your body. Breathe deeply, consistently. Feel the sensations in your body. Name the feelings that you notice. Accept the feelings and the sensations. Allow the thoughts and images to flow across your mind. Don't hold on to any one thing. Stay present.

Find the location in your body that is most alive with this wound, the place where you experience the most feelings and sensations that are related to this incident. You might find that memories of other moments that are associated may come to mind. If those memories are bigger and more central to your wound, follow them. If it feels like too much to handle, stay with the one you are on. Bring your breath with you to this location in the body. "Pendulate" back and forth as needed, like we did with the feelings. Observe, sense, and be present. Allow the emotions to flow. Be patient. This can be the extent you go to for the first few sessions. You are creating rapport with your wounded part, just as you did with your inner child. Creating safety and trust on both your parts. Eventually you can make more contact, like dipping your toe into the water slowly.

When you feel ready, you will begin to have more communication; it may come in words, sensations, or images. You may want to express the traditional Ho-opono-pono message, "I am sorry... Thank you for bringing this to my attention... Please forgive me... I love you..." in any way that feels meaningful. You might begin to have more awareness about when this part was first rejected by your family or yourself. Tell that part what you remember feeling at that time and how you see it now. You didn't know what else to do back then. But now you are learning how to soothe and connect with these parts.

See if you can bring that wounded part into your heart. Either imagine it or empower a pillow or stuffed animal to become that part for you to hold. Start where you can. Breathe, feel, witness. When you are ready, bring it into your arms. Connect with the Mother aspect of yourself. Be the mother you have always wanted, now for this part of you. Be compassionate. Tell that part something like, "I know it will take time for you to trust me, and that is ok. I am working on it. I am here now." You are bringing this part home to yourself. It is a powerful step. This takes practice and time, and it is worth every step. We are learning to love and accept our rejected parts. Anxiety melts in the face of this integration and redemption.

My client Sage is a 51-year-old savvy grandmother who has done some good work with herself. She is still very nervous about the Coming Home Process, but she shows up anyway. She chooses to address some early fears she has faced but not conquered. We work together to create safety and security while she calls in her resources. I guide her in focusing and pendulating as she rides the wave of feelings and sensations. I coach her on staying in touch with her Witness as she flows in and through the experience. She knows I am here with her. She grieves and screams and sobs. She mothers her wounded parts and forgives herself and others from her past. She frees herself of much pain. She is reclaiming her personal freedom and power. Her Heroine is rising.

In this chapter, we are deepening the process of self-care and responsibility for our entire physical, emotional, mental, and spiritual well-being. Just keep showing up for yourself one step at a time. As you grow your awareness slowly and lovingly, you will keep healing more places and feeling more powerful. Remember this is not about perfection, performance, and productivity; it is only about acknowledging, allowing, and awakening. Be gentle with yourself.

Main Messages:

1. The Heroine calls for compassion as our gift of courage for this Fear-Less path.
2. Calling in our resources and "pendulating" are strategies in the Coming Home Process.
3. Our ability to decrease our anxiety is related to our integration of our shadow parts.

Additional Tools of Discovery:

1. Dr. James Pennebaker's Writing Paradigm. This is a nice alternative way to work the Coming Home Process. Create a time and place to write with no disturbances for 15 minutes a day, and for three to four consecutive days. Promise yourself to follow through. You can write or type or tape record. Set a timer. Be honest and real. This is only for you. Write about your deepest emotions and thoughts about the most upsetting experiences in

your life. Let go. Free write. How is this experience related to who you would like to become? Who you have been? Who you are now? Focus on one area or many areas. Just write without thinking. Stop at the timer. Keep it or tear it or burn it; do whatever you feel pulled to do. This is a highly researched technique and a powerful tool for clearing out repressed emotional content(4).

2. Affirmations:

"I am courageous, compassionate, and kind with myself."

"I am slowly befriending my feelings more every day."

"I am willing and ready to integrate all parts of me slowly and lovingly."

PART FOUR

The Goddess

"The Goddess does not rule the world; She is the world.
Manifest in each of us ... in all her magnificent diversity."
– Starhawk

CHAPTER 12

———

The Spirit Dimension

"Turn within and seek the wisdom of your higher self. It is able to speak to us from the combined wisdom of our heart, mind, and spirit."

– Madison Taylor

The Goddess archetype reflects our spiritual nature as human beings. As women, the Goddess principle is our inherent connection with our own Soul and with the Creator. We may call this power greater than us by the name of God, Universe, Great Spirit, Divine Mother, Quan Yin, etc. The name is not as important as the way it connects us with this dynamic, universal consciousness of creation. Throughout this section, I will use different names for the God/Goddess. Feel free to substitute your preference as you read.

We are naturally born with this sacred nature and a capacity to be relational, caring, and expressive beings as women. We may not initially see the relationship between our spiritual identity and our issues with anxiety. Yet as multi-dimensional beings, we are wired for divine connection, and therefore we need to be curious for ourselves about how this part of us relates with our sense of self and our greater well-being. Our personal spirituality can be a game-changer on the Fear-Less Path where we can use our anxiety to grow, evolve, and actualize.

The Goddess principle within us is our intuition, our creativity, our expansiveness, our desire to serve, and our pull towards higher learning, spiritual growth, and self-actualization. Most of us have not been raised with this point of view here in the Western world, but in most indigenous cultures and Eastern spiritual paths, these concepts of the masculine and feminine principles are a well-known part of life. The Native American and South American traditions of Earth-based spirituality involve a daily connection with Mother Earth and Father Sky. People know they are a part of the entire web of life. In these cultures, when people suffer mentally, emotionally, or physically, it is considered a kind of soul sickness that requires a healing or soul retrieval ceremony. Suffering is considered a reflection of our disconnection from our bodies, soul, nature, and Great Spirit.

In modern times, the idea of being associated with your spiritual self has become less and less prioritized over the centuries. Historically, religion became known as the primary way people relate with their spiritual values. But for many, that is not enough. People do not always know they can cultivate their own personal relationship with the God/Goddess of their understanding. They don't experience the deeper connection they deeply want and need with the Divine. Our Western society denies this need for individuals to have their own personal spiritual relationship with God, and instead has it mediated through priests or other religious leaders. Our spiritual communion is not considered as important or valuable as money, power, and material goods. This is a crucial missing piece to our disconnection, which leads to anxiety for many people.

Many ancient cultures have predicted that during this time, there would be a return of the Universal Feminine energy of creation into our consciousness. As part of this change, chaos occurs as the old patriarchal way that is falling apart, fights to recover its power over the feminine by reducing our rights and access. Yet we are rising as women, as Goddesses. We are awakening. This is the Goddess in each of us, leading the way for our own personal healing and for humanity and Mother Earth.

In Part Four, we will explore our inner Goddess principle and her methods of helping us re-center ourselves, reduce our anxiety, and be the capable women we truly are. We look at the power of gratitude in shifting our mind, body, and spirit dimension to reduce anxiety. Then we recognize the essence of loving-kindness as a powerful teacher for learning authenticity and self-acceptance. In the last Spirit chapter, we learn about our empowerment through our divine connection that supports us in unveiling more of our True Selves.

CHAPTER 13

Gratitude

"Gratitude unlocks the fullness of life.... It turns denial into acceptance, chaos into order, confusion into clarity. It turns problems into gifts, failures into success and mistakes into important events. Gratitude makes sense of our past, brings peace for today, and creates a vision for tomorrow."

– Melanie Beattie

Gratitude is our ground zero in the Goddess Realm. It is the foundation from which our spiritual inspirations, values, and growth come. Gratitude means thankfulness, appreciation, or goodwill. It seems so simple, but it is so transformational. The Goddess aspect shows us how gratitude opens us to be more capable of perceiving life outside of our fearful minds and protected hearts. It becomes a doorway to clear our minds of fear and negativity and reveal our hearts with vulnerability to feel more joy, happiness, and peace.

Scientifically, gratitude meditation has been shown to significantly improve our ability to regulate our emotions, be more self-motivated and socially connect with others(1). The brain-heart-gratitude relationship has been verified to be quite meaningful, where an attitude of gratitude promotes improved mood, sleep, energy, self-efficacy, and spiritual well-being for people(2,3). This is powerful medicine, Goddesses. But we have not always known this.

Misconceptions of Gratitude

As children, we are taught to be grateful when we receive a gift from someone. We are obligated to say thank you and show appreciation. We do not understand the full meaning of it, just the mandatory response. We are not taught to wake up and feel gratitude for the day and for this gift of life and the chance to show up and live with awareness and joy. What a completely different concept of appreciating not only people and gifts, but life itself. This perception of gratitude is instinctive and embedded in indigenous and spiritual cultures. But in our modern world, we just haven't remembered the importance of it, until now. Let's first recognize a bit more how gratitude has been distorted and misguided in our Western culture.

Gratitude should only be considered when life is going "good." It is this negative perspective that says, "If I am struggling, what do I have to be happy and grateful about?" This attitude also can lead us to be envious, judgmental, and hateful of people we think have it better than us. We compare our painful insides to people's happy façades on the outside. This is our ego mind that keeps us stuck and focused on the problems as problems. Our hearts are shut-down, our minds have blinders on. Energy is not flowing. We are no longer grounded. We cannot experience life anew or see the multitude of choices we always have before us. This is how many of us unconsciously live, moving from one struggle or discontent to the next. We are only able to see what is not working in our life. It is such a huge loss to live this way. Millions of us do though, unintentionally. We do not even realize we have fallen in a hole.

Gratitude benefit us greatly in these moments of fear, panic, and anxiety. It is the ultimate diversion that can disengage us from our fear stories or "I'm not good enough" beliefs to look for the small things that are a blessing. It could be, "Well I lost my job, but I am grateful I have a roof over my head." This is where gratitude's capacity to see life differently happens. It gets us out of the hole and up on the mountain top, to perceive everything in another way.

However, if we think that feeling gratitude for small good things is being naïve or even superstitious, we will stay stuck. If we think we should feel guilty for not worrying about our problems, or we fear we're being irresponsible for feeling hopeful when things are hard, we will miss this opportunity. This is our anxiety believing we need to be worrying to be prepared for the next bad thing coming. But we know it isn't true. Worrying changes nothing. Suffering over our suffering keeps us in the hole. When we have an appreciative attitude for even the smallest of positive experiences in our lives, like a great cup of coffee or a beautiful sunset, it's like the blinds become opened in a dark room, allowing the light in. A small dose of gratitude can allow us to see how to address our challenges in ways we never thought of before. It sheds a new light on our world view.

Another misguided view is that we should always focus all our attention on others and wish well for them but not for ourselves. This is selfish. We learned that it's greedy to consider yourself at all. Here is how I see it: Selflessness is a higher-order principle we can live by once we are in a place of wellbeing and consciousness to offer that to people. But if we are struggling to get through the day with anxiety, pain, and struggle, we need to pull ourselves up and out of the hole first. Remember the airplane safety tactic? Put on your oxygen mask before your kids' mask. We, first, must heal and come into our wholeness before we can offer our care to others. The gift of gratitude fosters our capacity to open our hearts for ourselves and then for others.

Mary, a 57-year-old X-ray technician, has a protected heart, and for good reason. She has suffered in abusive relationships repeatedly in her life. She shuts her heart down to feel safer. I share the gratitude work with her in one session, and initially it is quite difficult for her to allow it in. She says her heart feels frozen. As Mary begins practicing gratitude daily on her own, she reports small but surprising changes. She is starting to be able to appreciate one small thing a day. Then she notices she is being a bit more kind with herself lately. It is fascinating and thrilling to me. Gratitude is like a deep underground river that gently moves us back into flow.

Your Bodhichitta Heart

Fear and anxiety tell us we should not open our hearts and feel gratitude every day, because it makes us too vulnerable; that our hearts are fragile and will break if we are open to the world. Having gratitude does open our hearts and expands our sense of trust and belonging in the world. However, we find out that our hearts are far from fragile when this happens. Our hearts are a dynamic vortex of energy charged up with love and light. We are actually stronger people when we open our hearts with consciousness. In Buddhism, the heart is a key spiritual center(4). They speak of Bodhichitta, meaning the "awakened heart," as our soft spot, when our hearts are broken open by life's suffering. This opening allows us to connect with others and love in an expanded, brilliant way. Our capacity to love increases from being broken wide open. Bodhichitta can transform the hardest, most closed-off hearts and the most fearful, closed minds. When we experience this tenderness, it links us to every human being on the planet. This is where healing and compassion happen. It is our woundedness that leads us to our wholeness and alliance with the web of life we are a part of.

Practice #1: Gratitude from the Heart

Create a quiet, undisturbed space. Ground and relax into your body. Breathe with awareness. Bring your Witness mind into the present moment. Set your intention for your experience; perhaps it's something like, "I want to be open to feeling gratitude." Then, while sitting or standing, bring your hands folded over the center of your chest to connect with the entire heart energy field, not just the heart organ. Open your consciousness to allow an awareness of gratitude to come up. Follow your intuition more than your thinking mind. Bring that image, sound, or thought of gratitude into focus. Notice the sensation of gratitude in your body. Imagine circulating it through your entire body through your bloodstream. Run it through your mind. Flow it into your heart. Be conscious of what you are experiencing, noticing energy or opening in the heart area, whatever is present. We might feel sadness or loss come up. That is natural. Acknowledge it and let it flow. Stay present. When you are near completion, you can choose to send out this gratitude as a prayer to someone you know, or to the world. Then come back into your body awareness. Breathe. Gently drop your arms and keep your eyes closed. Be still. Notice. Then open your eyes. It is nearly impossible not to smile afterwards.

The interesting evolution of gratitude is that, when we begin to see the world through grateful eyes, we notice how we can be accepting of life – not just how we want it, but on life's terms. It changes our perception to a larger-than-us perspective, as in the Neutral Mind. The Neutral or Witness Mind does not see in black or white. It always sees the whole bigger picture of how life is serving us, even when our ego says it is not what we ordered or wanted.

Practice #2: Journaling Gratitude for Your Challenges

Thankfulness for our challenges in life is another way to work with gratitude. How have your life struggles shaped you and helped you grow? What have they taught you about yourself? How have they shown you what is not working for you anymore? How does your anxiety do you a favor? You might become more aware of how anxiety is alerting you when you are ignoring a need, a boundary, or a feeling. Anxiety is always telling us, "Hey, pay attention!" How could you see your anxiety as a gift? How would your life change if you were grateful for your anxiety?

Take some time. Be present in your body and breathe. Be in your Witness. Begin to write from a non-thinking place. Read these questions, and then just write automatically without stopping for 15 minutes. Be honest and real. How do the messages from your anxiety help you show up for yourself? Has your anxiety made you smarter about what you need? Has it slowed you down from doing too much? Has it kept you from making bad choices and going against yourself? Does it help you love yourself? After you answer these questions, put the journal down. Breathe and notice how your body feels. Honor and thank yourself for being present with and for yourself, dear Goddess.

Leslie is a shy, bitter woman in her early 50s who is incredibly hard on herself every day. She secretly shames, blames, and criticizes herself in the way her mother did with her growing up – out of love, of course. As we search for a strategy to interrupt these patterns, I keep coming back to gratitude, despite her resistance. She eventually gives it a try. She starts practicing 2 minutes of self-love and gratitude with mirror work. When she comes to see me a few weeks later, she shares how she found herself saying "I am so grateful to you, Leslie!" over and over. It shocked her and opened her up. The grief and hurt can come out now for her to heal. She is able, at times, to be less obsessive and critical about herself. She can see how she is slowly showing up for herself in a new way. To celebrate, we did a minute of the happy dance together! It was a monumental shift, starting her down the path for healing and transformation.

Gratitude unfolds us to experience a more spiritual view of life. We can see how life's lessons come in all kinds of packages. In a study of patients with asymptomatic heart failure symptoms, the presence of gratitude was found to relate with people's reports of better sleep and mood, lower inflammation biomarkers, and improved spiritual wellbeing(3). It supports us be more aware of our choices in life, how we see things, and the way we want to show up for ourselves.

Gratitude connects us with our heart, and a perception that all of life is a gift: the good, the bad, and the ugly. It gives us new ways to let go of the past, stop worrying about the future, and be in the present, where the totality of possibilities lives. We can then develop our new perspectives about ourselves with loving-kindness.

Main Messages:

1. The Goddess teaches us gratitude to open our hearts and elevate our spirituality and wellbeing.
2. Bodhichitta, our wounded heart, allows us to feel a shared connection and compassion with others for the struggles and beauties of life.
3. Gratitude helps us honor the teachings that our anxiety has for us.

Additional Tools for Discovery

1. Alternate Nostril Breathing technique from Kundalini Yoga(5). This technique is used for balancing the right and left brain hemispheres and neutralizing our nervous systems. Keep the breath relaxed, deep, and full. Put your right hand near your face. As you begin to inhale, close off the right nostril with your thumb or index finger. Inhale through your left nostril. Then switch and close the left nostril and exhale out of the right nostril. Keep the left nostril closed and inhale through the right nostril long, slow, and deep. Then close off the right side and exhale out of the left. Begin the cycle all over again. Repeat it for at least three minutes. There is no maximum, so do the exercise until you get the desired effect. This breath is associated with calmness and stress- and anxiety-reduction(6).

2. Affirmations:

   "As I feel my gratitude, I am in the moment with an open heart."

   "I am grateful for the teachings of my anxiety."

   "My broken-open heart allows me to access my compassion for everyone's suffering."

   "I'm not alone."

CHAPTER 14

Loving Kindness

"The curious paradox is that when I accept myself just as I am,
then I can change."
– **Carl Rogers**

The Goddess represents our spiritual bravery and willingness to practice compassion, loving-kindness, and acceptance. When we are stuck in our anxiety, we cannot see the real us or the real world. Our fear beliefs tell us we are not worthy or good enough. We can completely lose touch with who we are. When we feel compromised, we tend to look outside of ourselves for a sense of power, attention, and approval. We might start people-pleasing to feel better in the moment, but it doesn't work in the long run. Looking outside of ourselves to be OK becomes another subtle form of self-abandonment and rejection. On the Fear-Less path, we have learned how gratitude can be used to soften our hearts. Self-acceptance is the next practice of embracing ourselves differently with kindness and respect.

Inviting Self-Acceptance

To learn self-acceptance is to see ourselves with the eyes of love. In Toltec tradition, one of the Four Agreements is that we always do our best. And our best is good enough on any given day, and it looks different every time. Doing our optimum is about starting where we are right now and practicing accepting all of us: our goodness, our pain, our light and our dark sides. This is the work we started in the mind dimension with our beliefs and continued in the body dimension by healing old wounds. Now, we will focus on accepting and holding space for all that we are and all that life teaches us.

In Tara Brach's work with trauma and Buddhist meditation, she calls the art of being with and regarding the present moment with compassion as being in "radical acceptance." She considers radical acceptance the gateway to healing our patterns and wounds and guiding us forward in our spiritual transformation(1). A recent study that uses radical acceptance as a tool for reducing avoidance of painful emotions found it to be remarkably helpful for people in decreasing their levels of shame, distress, and fear(2). This spiritual concept aligns with our practices in this Fear-Less path.

This view, of course, goes contrary to our ego's thinking that might say something like, "How can I accept myself yet, when I'm not good enough?" We tell ourselves, "Once I lose that weight or get that better job or someone loves me, then I can be good enough and accept myself." This is the paradox.

Our ego has a different agenda remember and therefore a disempowering definition. We truly are "enough" right now. We always were enough and we will always be enough. It is a constant and never changes. The way we cultivate this awareness is through focusing our attention and Witness consciousness on acceptance of ourselves.

Maitri Self-Love

Loving-kindness brings the "I am enough" feeling to a whole new level through different practices. In her book *The Places That Scare You*, Pema Chodron, a Tibetan Buddhist nun, writes about "Maitri" as a bodhichitta heart practice. She describes it as "placing our fearful mind in the cradle of loving-kindness." It is symbolized by the image of a mother bird caring and protecting her baby chick until it is capable to fly on its own. In this image, we are both the mature responsible mother and the desperate, raw, and needy baby bird. This way, we learn to embrace and love all parts of ourselves.

It is time to get out of the black-and-white view of life and see the acceptable, large gray zone of reality. We start with focusing on loving and accepting ourselves. Then we move to accepting others as they are. Eventually, we can love all that life is, without bias. We can recognize how life is perfect in each moment just as it is – from our neutral mind, of course. The beauty is that current loving-kindness research shows how this practice is also applicable in reducing depression, anxiety, anger, and other challenging mental health symptoms in various populations(3,4).

Joan, a kind 57-year-old woman, shares how she has always had a negative body-image of herself. Her anxiety revolves around her self-loathing. She can't be with girlfriends without comparing her body to theirs and self-shaming. I offer loving-kindness as a therapeutic approach to her challenges. She is surprisingly willing to start practicing with mirror work. She begins building a new connection with her body as a part of her instead of as an object. She is cautioned to not permit herself to use the mirror against herself, letting her Inner Critic take over. She recently told me that she is beginning to feel compassion for herself and her body for the first time ever. She feels how her body suffers every time she judges it harshly. She is able to locate a small bit of acceptance. She continues practicing loving-kindness towards herself and her body as a major goal of her healing path. Her anxiety is decreasing more and more as her self-love gets bigger than her self-hate. Cheers, Goddess! What a tribute to the body.

Practice #1: Accepting Yourself

Connect with your Witness Self. Observe how you feel in your body. Breathe and feel your body breathing. Now, pick one physical aspect you dislike or one shameful feeling in your body. Recognize all the beliefs and old stories about how this part is not OK. Now distance yourself from the stories. Imagine them moving three miles away in front of or behind you. They still might try and get your attention, but they are like tiny fleas on the horizon now.

Now, open your bodhichitta heart and send love to that unloved part right now. Put your hands on the relating body part. Feel compassion for the years of rejection and judgment of this part. Now tell this part that it is doing the best it can, as are you. Consciously breathe into this area with heartfelt compassion. Relax your body. Imagine releasing all the shame, pain, and hurt in a flow of energy running down your body and into the Earth. Then, focus on emanating loving-acceptance through your hands to this part of you. Acceptance that says, "I may not like you as you are, but I accept you. You are a part of me," or "I am willing to learn how to accept you as you are." Start where you are. Keep holding that vision of acceptance. Allow whatever feelings arise; let them flow. No judgment. Stay in your Witness Self. Notice how this body part responds to you accepting it at whatever level you could. Recognize any release, energy shifting, or feelings moving. If this area feels numb, that's normal. Stay with that. Whatever shows up is perfect. Be patient. Close with honor and gratitude to yourself for showing up.

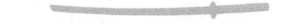

"Authenticity is the daily practice of letting go of who we think we are supposed to be and embracing who we are."

– Brené Brown

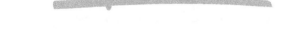

Getting Real

As we evolve our acceptance of ourselves, we naturally begin to be more authentic in our lives. Authenticity is the ability to be our True Self, who we are at a soul level, behind the mask of our ego. When we value ourselves, we lose the need to focus on other people to approve of us or to feel like we belong. We no longer need to sacrifice ourselves by denying our needs and wants. Our anxiety may still worry about us upsetting people, but it will fade away slowly. As we gain this stronger sense of self, we start feeling more at home in ourselves, our bodies, and our minds. We have less of a need to have everyone be our friend, and we accept being our own best friend. We can be more honest and truthful in our relationships with ourselves and with others. It is such a huge freedom. And, of course, it relates directly with reducing our anxiety.

We realize that being authentic is not only favorable for ourselves and our self-esteem, it genuinely evolves our relationships in a way we couldn't expect. People respect us more because we are self-respecting. People develop their own boundaries, as we are doing. There is more integrity within our relationships instead of codependency. It is a serious win-win outcome.

Katie, a dear 30-year-old mother, who grew up with a mentally ill single mother, sees me to address her postpartum anxiety. Her stress revolves around her mother, who still relies on her. Yet her mother refuses to care for herself or accept any treatment. Katie has been full of anxiety her whole life, feeling in charge but helpless. She loves her mom and she recognizes that it is more than she can handle, when she can barely manage her own self-care. Authenticity is the open window to see the truth of the situation through new eyes. Katie sees how her mom is choosing her path and ignoring her own needs. She, first, accepts the reality of who her mom is and where she is stuck in herself. Then she faces her own limits and responsibilities to herself, her child, and her family now. Katie gets a perspective of her own values, needs and choices. She realizes that she can love her mother, and it doesn't mean she has to keep being responsible for her. She can respect her mother's choices and have her own integrity. Her anxiety has reduced tremendously. She accepts her mother now and she takes better care of herself and her family in a whole new way. Impressive work, Goddess.

Practice #2: Trying On Authenticity

Take out your journal. Connect with your Witness self. Notice your breath, your body awareness. For 5-10 minutes, write about the recent dynamics in three primary relationships in your life. It can be with partners, friends, bosses, children, or parents. Ask yourself to honestly notice where in each relationship you are withholding your truth about something you need or want. Be real. Keep your ego out of it. Stay present in the moment and relaxed in your body. If feelings come up, honor them and let them pass. See if you can fully acknowledge what isn't working for you in these relationships, without judging yourself or the other person. Then write any values that are being disrespected or disregarded by yourself or the other person, that are possibly contributing to you feeling not OK in those relationships. Just allow yourself to take in what you are becoming aware of.

Then write one action step you could take in each relationship as a baby step towards re-aligning yourself with your values and inner truth. Remember, you may not get what you want from others, but you need to ask anyway and see what's possible, especially if it is a relationship that matters a lot to you. Take the next few weeks to practice these action steps and communicate more of what you want in each relationship. Notice what happens internally in your mind and body and externally in the relationship. You can make a huge difference in developing your maturity by being more authentic. Relationships can truly transform when both parties are willing to show up this way.

Roseann, a 48-year-old wonderful character of a woman, is a caretaker in her relationships. She loves it and hates it. Secretly, she wants to be cared for. Once she realizes why she does this, she understands why she is anxious and agitated most of the time. She does a lot of journal work for a few weeks before she feels brave enough to speak up in her relationships about her truth. Some people were very open and loving, while others were angry with her. She is seeing she needs to decide which relationships support her wellbeing and which ones she will let go of. She is prioritizing herself for the first time and creating a better life. Anxiety is releasing slowly. It's beautiful to see Roseann prioritize and care for herself and know the significance.

Learning how to love, accept, and be true to ourselves takes time, spiritual bravery, and vulnerability. It is also life-changing and life-affirming. Aligning with ourselves in this way makes it hard for anxiety to stick around, because we will know the message loud and clear about what we need. And then we take action and do it. You got this, Goddess!

Main Messages:

1. The Goddess helps us learn through loving-kindness, to accept ourselves in an authentic, loving way.

2. Loving-kindness through the Maitri practice heals our judgment and disconnection from ourselves and others.

3. Authenticity is our greatest gift to ourselves and each other.

Additional Exercises:

1. Formal Maitri-Meditation(5). Center and ground yourself. Be present in your Witness. You will offer loving-kindness in seven stages. A general offering is, "May I have peace and happiness." You serve it to yourself out loud and with conscious focus from your heart. Then, say it out loud and apply it to 1) your loved ones, 2) your friends, 3) "neutral" people in your life, 4) those who irritate you, 5) all of the above as a group, and 6) all beings throughout time and space. Go at your own pace and feel the experience in your body, your heart, and your soul. Allow emotions to be acknowledged as they come and go. Stay awake to all the nuances of feelings, sensations, energy, and imagery. Journal about your experience. After practicing it a few times in a calm state, try it when you are at a 1-4 on your anxiety scale and see what happens.

2. Affirmations:

"I accept all of me today, no matter what."

"I feel loving-kindness toward myself and others more every day."

"I am loving more of who I am and letting go of what no longer serves me."

CHAPTER 15

━━━━━

Divine Connection

"Awaken to your own internal power, to your own connection to
the Divine and act on what you are inspired to do."

– Joe Vitale

Our Divine connection is the next step of the Goddess
principle on this Fear-Less Path. The Goddess continues
to guide us toward exploring our own spirituality and its
relationship to our anxiety. Having faith or spiritual bearing is
our invisible thread to our intuitive knowing. It is a deep inner
trust, without reservation, in a perception of a power greater
than us, which is intrinsic. Metaphorically, it is like being a
drop of water within in the vast ocean; spirituality gives us a
context for our life. When we are lost in anxiety, we lose this
context and can feel alone and disconnected from people we
love, and ourselves. We can feel deserted.

Why Be Faith-Connected?

This concept of Divine relationship may be related with religion for you, but that is only one way to look at it. There are a hundred different paths to reach God consciousness through religion, spiritual practice, meditation, yoga, ecstatic dance, Qi-gong, art, music, and countless other modalities. We are allowed as humans to explore which ways resonate the most for us at any given time. It is my experience that our spiritual path grows and evolves over time as we develop in our creativity and consciousness. What I am addressing here is our daily personal connection with Spirit that reflects in our lifestyle, as well. Our spiritual beliefs give us direction with our values, our decisions, and our sense of purpose. This part of us is essential for our growth, our greater well-being, and our mental health. A recent study affirms that our existential need for meaning and our spiritual need for release from despair, shame, and guilt are imperative for our mental health and well-being(1). Therefore, it is necessary to find ways we can receive that inspiration, love, and presence in Goddess connection.

A recent article acknowledges that human spirituality has been excluded from our Western ideas of health and the healing process, to our detriment. It cites Carl Jung, saying, "Every crisis is a spiritual crisis." The article writes "Stress is the threat of unresolved anger and fear, which chokes our human spirit and life force"(2). Anything that affects us mentally also impacts us emotionally, physically, and spiritually as well. We need to start applying this holistic perspective to our health, lifestyle and overall wellbeing to adequately address our anxiety.

Another study found that women with a well-developed psycho-spiritual sense of wellbeing could cope more effectively with a diagnosis of terminal illness and find meaning in the process than women without this wellbeing(3). Having a spiritual connection can help us feel we are part of a bigger context which vastly supports our whole self. Even though we cannot prove the existence of God/Goddess, does believing in a God/dess serve us more than not believing? Does it feel more comforting? Does it help us stay aligned with our true values? Does it give us focus or purpose that helps carry us through our life challenges and anxiety to the other side of calmness?

The realm of our inner Goddess is our opportunity to widen our scope of what are acceptable, supportive, spiritual modalities for us. There are a multitude of ways to feel held and guided by Source. In Chapter 3, I shared my journey about exploring different paths that were purposeful and meaningful for me. In my 50s, it became very important to me to study divine feminine and embodiment practices. I fell in love with the Divine Mother, which felt like a reunion with feminine self and my feminine lineage that I had lost as a young girl. Reconnecting helped me heal my relationship with my mother who had passed away and recover my own feminine wisdom I had let go of in the face of pleasing the masculine patriarchy. Now I merge all the teachings that have assisted me into a method that feels most honoring and sacred for me.

It is all about giving ourselves permission, which is what empowerment means. We can authorize ourselves to find what we need and want and incorporate it into our lives. We are allowed to expand our spiritual beliefs in ways that may strengthen, embody, and cultivate our relationship with our own souls and God. Having a Divine connection can give us the ability to relate with our own personal power in an ethical, valuable, and beautiful way.

Practice #1: Recognizing Your Ego Obstacles

Here are some ways that the ego can get in our way. Give yourself permission to explore the thoughts and feelings that come up and write them down if you choose. There is no judgment here, only awareness and choices. You might feel guilty for considering going outside of a religious faith that you grew up with or are currently connected to. This is a very common challenge. Anxiety tells us we are being bad and we are betraying our faith. I ask you, if exploring and trying new ways to connect with the Creator of your understanding increases your faith, joy, and happiness, how is that a bad thing? Why does it upset others when you relate with that God in this way? And if it's a problem with your community, how does it feel to be told that your precious personal relationship with Goddess can only look a certain acceptable way? Just be open to your inner knowing. Another part of this confusion may be the idea that you must choose only one way to love and connect with God. You must to be a Christian, a Sufi, a Jew, a Muslim, or a Pagan. In my view, they all lead to the same place. Can you let yourself wonder about this and find your truth inside?

The other obstacle you might perceive is that you must choose a path already created by others. That is a common misperception by people who have grown up in a particular structured faith. We are co-creators here. It's your choice to create what works for you. Even if it's made piecemeal of parts of many paths in your own unique format. Your personal relationship with Source, Higher Self, God/Goddess is yours and yours alone. It is your call and your co-creation.

Lena, age 29, grew up in a strict, religious home that requires her to participate in religious services whether she wants to or not. It creates a lot of pain and confusion for her. She loves God. She just doesn't relate to her parents' religious choice. When she finally came out as a lesbian, it has been torture since. Her parent's judge her and try to "fix" her. Lena has chosen to distance herself just to survive. She cut off spiritually for a long time as a result. When she came to see me about her anxiety, it became clear we needed to explore this spiritual part. She was relieved to hear the perspective that it is her choice about how she connects with the Divine. That alone created space for her anxiety to change. On a recent visit, she came in sheepishly smiling and said that she found a version of God that works for her. Her God/Goddess is a Fairy Godmother character out of a Disney movie because she feels loved, supported, and accepted with it. It totally works for her. I congratulated on her bravery and persistence in finding her truth and a spiritual relationship that respects and loves her.

Practice #2: Choose a Faith Place to Start

This is a practice, not a dedication. This is your experiential inquiry of what may work for you. I want you to sit quietly with your feet on the floor. Be present and conscious. Set your intention about what you would like for yourself from this exercise. Set a space of protection energetically as well, asking for only energies of highest good can come. Think about what concept of the Larger-Than-You Creator you want to visit right now. It might be Buddha, God, Archangel Michael, Hera the Greek Goddess, Divine Mother, Jesus, Great Spirit, etc. Be open. See what your heart says. Once you have focused in on one thing, imagine feeling a thread of light running up your spine, continuing above your head. This your light, your being. Imagine a thread coming down from the Larger-Than-You Creator. Let the threads meet and connect. What does that feel like? Does your body respond? Notice if you feel any emotions? Allow your experience to unfold organically. Receive without evaluating or judging. Each time you practice allow yourself to go deeper into the communication and connection and see what happens. Notice how it feels afterwards.

Why Divine Connection Serves Anxiety

Most spiritual paths say that God/Goddess, Creator, Great Spirit is always there for us, whether we are conscious of it or not. The important thing here is defining what "being there for us" means. Does it mean Goddess is protecting us from life's dangers? Or does it mean that Goddess is with us on our life journey whether it is easy or hard? Many spiritual paths talk about the Divine Creator being respectful of our personal will and choice to suffer in our lifetime. They say the door is always there, but it's up to us to open it and ask for assistance. It is only then that guidance will come in some form, and not always in the way we want it. So, if I choose to feel alone and stay feeling sorry for myself, Source will respect that. It does not see suffering as good or bad, it is just how we grow. But if I wake up in the morning and I ask for support and assistance in staying on my path, will that Source will show up for me? This is another exploration.

Diane, age 33, is an atheist who struggles with panic attacks. She has a Zen meditation practice that has supported her for a few years. Her mother died recently, and that's when her panic attacks started. Among other work, we choose to explore her spirituality. I ask her about this concept of asking for spiritual support and how that could possibly work for her in this grief process. She leaves this session doubtful, but says she is willing to sit with it. She comes back in the next week looking excited. First she says she has not had a panic attack in a week. Then she reveals how she experienced the most loving motherly connection with a Female Goddess she asked to help her with dealing with her mother's death. She started to tear up. It was beyond moving. Now does this mean she must stop being atheist? No. Does it mean she is a pagan now? No. Is she allowed to give herself this support no matter what anyone else thinks about it? Yes. Welcome to personal freedom, Goddess.

Practice #3: Asking for Support

Do this practice when you have a good 15 minutes alone. Sit in your personal space or in nature. Bring your awareness to the Witness Self. Feel your body. Notice your breath. Bring your focus inside of you. Feel what is present in your heart, body, and mind. Intuitively imagine what connection you need right now for i.e., the most loving, nurturing support or whatever is most important to you right now. Allow an opening as we did in the above exercise. Give yourself permission to broaden how the

Divine can show up right now, what could happen? It may be one of the spiritual names I offered before or it may be a sacred animal, a messenger, or a symbol like a triangle or a tree. Trust yourself and your intuition.

Settle in with one image now. Open your heart and ask for what you need from this reflection of God/Goddess. Something like "Thank you for coming to aid me. I am having a hard time with my fears, can you stand by me and help see me through them?" Whatever you need to say is what is best for you. Have a conversation of sorts. Just trust yourself and allow yourself to receive support. Notice your breath, your body sensations, and your response to this experience. At first, it can feel almost silly and fake. That is just the ego mind. Stay with it and give it time to develop into a calming, peaceful moment. Take time to integrate it and maybe journal it.

Another purpose of Divine connection is to help us to step back and see the bigger picture of life. How can we benefit from stepping out of our small life and our ego's blinders that keep us trapped in our little view of life? What could be different if we could sit on a mountain top like an eagle and view the world from there? People are now just tiny little dots. We see how we are all trying to find our way. Is it especially harder for us? Probably not too much different than the other billion people out there. A little perspective helps us see how we are more similar than different. This can shift us into a new perspective, not only for our personal world but with humanity. The bigger view gives us a reminder of our larger connection with everything, and for many, it confirms their spiritual experience of the Infinite. Our anxiety can keep us feeling separate and disconnected from others. We can get lost in our own troubles, especially if we don't ask for help. Spirituality and Divine connection help us be more aware of the All-One-Ness that is present, whether we see it or not, as well.

Practice #4: The Bigger Picture

When you are struggling with a rough time, this practice can pull off your blinders and allow you to see quite differently. Sit and center yourself. Dis-invite the ego mind. Be in your Observer self. Face the challenges with your heart open and your body grounded. Acknowledge your pain without judgment. Name the feelings and the sensations that are present in your body. Allow them to be, without resistance or indulging. Now, imagine you are looking down at the little you that is this struggling human being from way up high on a cloud. Feel the compassion for that little you.

Now imagine all the hundreds of people near you that you notice are also struggling. Keep backing up, and now see the thousands of people. Observe how impersonal it all is when we see everyone going through life. It is not just about me and my anxiety. It is everyone on their life journey. And we are all in the same boat, no matter our skin color, our faith, our gender, our orientation, our economic status, or our age. Life is everywhere and we are all in it, doing the best we can.

From this eagle eye view, we can see the possibilities of life more easily than when we are stuck with blinders, focusing on the problem. The choice to know the All-One perspective instead of the I-am-A-lone is one of the possibilities. This All-One state of being, ironically, is the belonging we are often looking for when we give up parts of ourselves to fit in or people please with others. In this state, however, you are uniquely perfect and there is no need to change yourself at all. You belong, no matter what. You are a part of the whole always. Anxiety shifts with this perspective.

When we have this bigger view, we can often be inspired to go help others who need support. This is powerful not only for the people who get to feel cared about, it also invites us to our share our gifts of who we truly are. And when we are of service, we get to embody the feeling and knowing that we are a part of the world. We get to reconnect with life's meaning in a new way. Serving others also combats anxiety because we feel useful instead of useless. It gives us focus on something other than our self and our struggle. This opens us to see what is possible, what we have to be grateful for, or to notice life can be precious and rich, even when it is hard.

Frida, a 40–year-old woman, suffers with severe anxiety and panic attacks. She has been in many abusive relationships. Life has not been easy for her. She works hard just to get through the day. She is quite resistant. I realize she does not feel capable or worth much in herself, so getting help is challenging her. I decide it may be encouraging for her to experiment with Divine connection as a way to see her own value. We practice meditation in the session, with me guiding her and inviting her to connect with her Source. She reports afterwards, "I feel some peace, and can get a break from my crazy thoughts." They are there but quieter. After a few months of her practicing in sessions, the panic attacks start to recede.

Months later, she tells me she is beginning to feel more calm and compassionate with herself. She is noticing how she is less critical of herself and doesn't know how it is happening. I tell her this is what can happen with spiritual connection and meditation. It expands our experience of ourselves, and what is false, or no longer serving us, starts to fall away. She also feels more resourced and less alone in her life, even though nothing on the outside has changed. She is practicing self-care, which is novel. She is accepting her self-worth, which is momentous. Her anxiety comes as an occasional visitor and she knows how to work with it. Now she is starting to volunteer at the local domestic shelter for women. She is becoming a beautiful butterfly in her life. It is absolutely amazing.

Current research reflects the incredible positive impact of meditation not only for our physical health and immune system(4), but also for our ability to do our self-care and reduce our anxiety(5). Meditation has a potent impact on our ability to stay centered and connected to the Divine throughout our day. There are many transformative layers of growth that meditation can take us through when we are ready.

This practice of our spiritual connection is a process, not a one-and-done. So be patient and be loving. Most of all, be open to your own inner guidance in the process. It is about getting to know yourself and experiencing life from the inside-out. There are a million ways to encounter our Divine connection, so have fun and notice how your anxiety falls away.

Main Messages:

1. Through spirituality and divine connection, the God/ Goddess empowers us with a sense of meaning and purpose.

2. Allowing ourselves to feel resourced and a part of something larger than us decreases our anxiety.

3. Having a bigger picture of life offers us the uplifting experience of our interconnection with humanity and life on the planet.

Additional Tools of Discovery:

1. Establish a Sacred Space and Time. Create your own place for Divine connection in your life. It can be a corner of a room where you have a place to sit, with an altar or a candle. Put special objects or pictures of meaningful teachers, loved ones, or yourself there. Let it evolve and grow. Set a time of day or at least an amount of time you will give yourself daily to spend in your sacred space. Mindfully stretch, pray, do yoga, dance, do tai chi, meditate, sit quiet. Try anything. Try everything. See what you love and do it. Pick the time and do something every day for 90 days, then see what you notice.

2. Affirmations:
   "I am divinely connected and powerful today."
   "I am resourced and held in love and light."
   "I open to guidance and love from Source."

PART FIVE

"Change isn't always easy, but with purposeful practice,
any old habit can be replaced with a way of being we would
recommend to those we love."

– Bill Crawford

CHAPTER 16

Distractions and Detours

"Success doesn't come from what you do occasionally,
it comes from what you do consistently."
– Maria Forleo

You have come through the reading and worked with some of the practices and hopefully you've experienced a shifting in your perceptions, understanding, and awareness of your anxiety. The more you bring these teachings into your life, the more you can hone your skills for getting to the heart of what your anxiety is showing you. In this way, anxiety becomes our personal aide in helping us stay attentive to ourselves on all levels – physically, emotionally, mentally, and spiritually. It becomes our warning signal. Every life path has blessings and challenges. And no matter how powerful a program is, there will always be obstacles that we must face. It's as if we are on a boat on the ocean. Storms will come. The waves will warn us and start knocking us about. How do we be alert, and prepared and stay in the boat when the storms of life come?

Distraction and Re-Tracking

Distraction comes from our ego, which is threatened by the truth of who we are, which is much bigger and more powerful than the ego can ever be. Our lower brain and ego will be unsupportive of our desire to change things up and evolve. Remember, sameness is safety for the ego. As we discussed in the introduction, it is essential for you to keep paying attention to which part of yourself you're listening to. Which are the beliefs that support you and your right to live in peace? Which beliefs would be best for you to have up front and central for you? This is a question we need to keep asking ourselves every day. Otherwise, the old habits of the mind will knock us off our boat, like waves and distract us from what we want.

Getting distracted is normal, we know. We want to get some work done, and the kids need us. We want to get to the gym more, but we need to clean the house. You see how life is constant, ever-flowing with the next wave? How can we stay focused, afloat, and connected with what is important to us? What helps you stay on track? Because it's easy to just toss this book aside and go back to life as it is and allow the anxiety to continue to run you. Plenty of people do it every day. You can give up and lose sight of the pain that brought you here in the first place. Or you can focus on the pain of the anxiety and get weary. And then you fall back in the hole and don't even realize it.

What we focus on grows. In this program, we learn to observe and acknowledge the pain, anxiety, the fear stories, and the physical sensations and let them pass. We don't resist and we don't hyperfocus. Be devoted to yourself. Stay with me here, and let's strategize a plan to keep you on track and on the boat.

This path is not just about becoming skilled with these practices to stop anxiety. It is more transformational and meaningful than that. It is ultimately about living with awareness, happiness, and freedom to be your True Self. It is about being who you came here to be. How we prioritize our time, attention, and energy on what matters is essential. Like a carrier pigeon, there will be stops along the way, but you know the ultimate direction to keep flying to get home. With your anxiety and your self-care practices, you need to use your carrier pigeon skills and stay the course.

How can you stay connected with what matters? How can you remain attached to who you are? By immersing yourself into the program and gathering the resources that can help. There is a saying in recovery, "Don't wait until you are losing it, HALT!" We learn to pay attention to whether we are allowing ourselves to get too hungry, too angry, too lonely, or too tired (HALT). When we are there, we have already gone past the point of being helpful to ourselves or others. The trick is to manage your self-care and stop pushing with perfectionism, so you see it coming and act differently to avoid the HALT place altogether. This can be a good reminder to keep an eye on yourself.

Becoming devoted to your self-care and embodiment can be one of your greatest tools in the beginning. If you are keeping self-care and body awareness as a regular practice in any form at least 2-3 days a week, you will be increasing your ability to stay more present and real with yourself. If you start taking two or three days off from any self-care practice, you will begin sliding down the proverbial hill back into life as normal again, with the misery, anxiety, and pain. Your ego will take charge and you will forget why you wanted to try something new.

Gina, an intelligent 33-year-old woman, struggles with staying on track. It is a challenge for her to remember her practices, let alone do them. Once she became a parent, it was that much harder. Her anxiety and fear also escalated. She works on being honest and more real with herself to stay aware of the consequences of slipping off track. She slips and then she gets back on track. This is her greatest achievement, to not give up on herself like she did in the past just because she slips up. Now, she asks for support from me and other resources in her life to get back on track again and again. She can re-center herself faster and more often than ever before. She still knows that life without anxiety running the show is the goal and her self-care and practices need to be prioritized for her to keep moving forward. She does her best and it is good enough. She found that her greatest gift is her discipline to not give up on herself.

We are all going to fall off track and get distracted. But the more we pay attention, the more we will notice before, during and after that happens and then we can make a new choice. We need to be courageous and forgiving, and get back up on our feet and keep going, doing our best. It will never be about perfection and doing it "right" all of the time. Doing our best includes screwing up, owning it, and getting back on track. It just takes practice and compassion to know that in life we all fall and get back up again, all the time. It's part of growing up and learning.

What Matters

Our immediate gratification culture is a real distraction problem. We want the fix-it pill, and we do not want to have to work for it. We think we can bypass the "real" work of growing up as a human being. But how many people do you know who have all the toys that society says they need to be happy, and yet they are miserable, unhappy people? Our Western culture says it values family, responsibility, equality, and kindness but it teaches us a completely opposite message through advertisement, media, politics, and how money is allocated. It can be very confusing and hard to hold on to what matters most in our culture. Here we are trying to create positive changes for ourselves, and we have to stay conscious and vigilant about the contrary messages we can get side-tracked with so easily from the outside world. This is where a daily routine of something; silence, prayer, stretching, meditation, or breathing practice can help us clear out the unhelpful thoughts, emotions, and energy we pick up everyday without knowing it.

Another distraction can be the next great fad. Our culture loves sensationalizing new ideas, to promote and sell things, like juicing or Zumba or even mindfulness. In his book, *Spiritual Materialism*, Trungpa Rinpoche speaks to this way our culture can turn anything of great value, essence, and importance into a fad. It has taken the thousand-year-old powerful practice of yoga as a consciousness path and turned it into a materialistic clothing competition. It is frightening, really. Losing perspective of what really matters can happen so easily. How can we stay real about our potential life transformation with this Fear-Less path and keep it the most important thing in our life?

This program, your ego might say, will get boring, and we don't have time for it. But we have two hours to watch TV, and one hour for Facebook, and an hour and a half for the coffee shop.... There are more fun things to entertain us than these practices. This is what our culture has brainwashed us with: to be easily distracted, bored, and seeking entertainment as a source of happiness. However, that kind of happiness will never last. All the yogis and sages have known this for thousands of years. Happiness is a state of mind and perception and choice. It isn't a destination.

A different form of interference our ego loves to employ is to become the continual seeker. We just want to keep learning new things but never apply anything. So, we just move from one thing to the next, searching for the pleasure of the experience, but missing the heart of transformation that is available. When we get caught in this self-help cycle or spiritual window shopping, we will always fall back to the status quo of our default ego system, staying unhappy, stuck, and powerless. It just, unfortunately, will not do the trick.

We can also get caught in a fear story about how we don't have enough time or money to invest in ourselves and what is good for us. Yet we spend hours watching TV and we waste countless dollars on unimportant things every day; $5 on coffee, $12 on lunch out, $20 on that video game. It keeps us in the place we already are. If we want to be in a different place in ourselves and our lives, we need to see the bigger picture, beyond the moment. If we keep doing the same thing, we will keep getting the same results.

We need to figure out what is most valuable to us. Is life without anxiety important to us or not? This simple question is compelling enough to help us get back on track. Like anything, a new behavior/habit in our life requires a level of commitment to our true needs and wants. If Sherri wants to advance in her career as a nurse, she must advance her learning and skills. That means more school, more studying, and more practicing. If Josie wants to become healthy after having cancer, she needs to learn what works best for her to eat, how much sleep she needs, what supplements are helpful, and which exercise regimes work best for her. It is not just one thing. It is multiple things that she needs to learn and put into place one a time.

One step at a time is all we can do. Each change requires this attention, self-devotion, and bigger picture. Otherwise, we wake up and wonder, "What am I doing all this for again? I forgot." And our ego takes over to sabotage us and keep us small and stuck again. It is just one step at a time.

Drastic Detours

Detours are the life events that we allow to capture all our attention. Detours can look like life hitting the fan: losing a job, a relationship ending, or getting sick. We no longer care enough for ourselves because something challenging is happening, we lose our footing. We default to old beliefs that say it is more important to get stressed, worried, and upset about this problem than to practice my tools. This is us caught in the storm of life and anxiety, on our boat in the middle of a huge storm. And believe me, when this storm comes, this is when we need to have our skills in place, or we can get blown so far off course by the storm. We can fall out of the boat and get lost swimming in circles. We can't see or think clearly. It feels like everything is lost, but it's not. We can use our skills and calm down, breathe and find our boat and wait out the storm. For some people, detours can take years to recover from and get back to the place they were.

Janie, a 36-year-old professional, faced a serious detour after she worked in this program. She had finished the nine-week program and was doing her practices regularly. It was making a big difference for her quality of life and supporting her personal recovery with alcohol. Her anxiety was improving. She thought she had enough support in her life and decided not to continue with the ongoing coaching program. A month later, she lost her job and her anxiety escalated and took hold of her. She fell back into old bad habits and pain. She didn't reach out. She got isolated, and lost. It took her about a year and a half for her to pull out of it. That's when I saw her and she told me what happened. It was heartbreaking to hear it. It can happen so easily to anyone if we are not prepared and practiced in our program.

When you have a daily practice in place, it becomes the ground that helps you weather the storm. It keeps you more aligned with yourself than with fear. It allows you to use those new skills and stay on track despite the storm. I believe my daily practice helped me get through my cancer the way I did. Emotionally, mentally, spiritually and physically, I know it was one of my major resources.

Another detour we can take is when we stop caring about ourselves and get apathetic. We let a hard day become a hard life, and our ego takes over and says, "Why bother trying?" We all feel this at times for a few hours or days maybe. But when it collapses your life into a dark cloud and you accept that this is how it will always be, this is big trouble. The backlash of your ego and old habits are trying to take over and sabotage not just the new skills but literally disempower you altogether. A mutiny, we could say. This detour is dangerous. This requires a 911 call to your nearest friend or relative. This means getting some immediate help, either from family or professionals. Do not wait. Do it now.

Making a Plan

Detours are dangerous. We can regress in our abilities when we let our fear take over. We need to know how precious this chance is to wake up and live differently. What an opportunity this is to be your True Self, be the light you are, and live with happiness, peace and freedom. Having enough resources is the key for any change. Make a solid plan and support yourself to arrive at your destination like the carrier pigeon. You deserve it. We all do. It is our birthright. Make sure this happens by making a solid plan for the next 12-18 months at least. This includes who your support is and what your resources are, inside and out. This includes your plan B, just in case plan A doesn't get you there.

This is an empowering path to Fear-Less-ness. It has all the tools and strategies that can support you, but there will always be obstacles. Most people have a much better chance to succeed if they work with me, because I have walked this path and faced the dangers of getting off track. I also carry with me the knowledge and the lineage of a handful of spiritual paths that keep me grounded and able to help others on this path. Consider your options and meditate with them. Give yourself the best shot at getting what you want for yourself and your life. Do it now. If not now, when? You are worth it.

CHAPTER 17

━━━━━

Conclusion

"When you recover or discover something that nourishes your
Soul and brings joy, Care enough about yourself to make room
for it in your life."

– Jean Shiboda Bolen

Y̲ou made it. Getting acquainted with the program is
the most important first step. You showed up. You are
courageous and powerful. Let's do a quick review of what you
have learned.

In Part Two, we reconnected with our Queen principle
to have power over our Mind by reclaiming our self-worth
from our Inner Critic. We developed the Witness awareness to
acknowledge our fear stories and allow them to pass by without
getting hooked by them. Then we learned in the Dignity
chapter about self-respect and responsibility and how this helps

us create our boundaries and our self-care practices. In the Sovereignty chapter, we applied the Toltec Four Agreements as a tool for self-awareness and changing our mental habits. We inventoried our beliefs and re-assigned our advisory committee.

In Part Three, we experienced the necessary tools of embodiment and breath in applying the gift of reverence for our loyal bodies. We learned that being grounded decreases anxiety. We explored the role of feelings, sensations, and "pendulating" in the Wisdom chapter. The Courage chapter informed us of the importance of our internal and external resources in the recovery of our wounded parts in the Coming Home Process.

Part Four, the Goddess, presented Spirit as the last critical domain in our healing work with anxiety. We experienced the power of gratitude in releasing anxiety and cultivating our wellbeing. In the Loving-Kindness chapter, we recognized the importance of self-acceptance and authenticity as the keys for loving-kindness towards ourselves and for others. In the Divine Connection chapter, we explored the fundamental role of faith and spirituality in feeling resourced and interconnected with others. We saw how the bigger picture view helps us be more kind, open, and appreciative at any given moment. This reinforces our calm acceptance and prevents our fearful anxiety from being our filter through which we see the world.

It is my wish that you don't delay and that you stay the course, like the homing pigeon, to receive and integrate these teachings as your own in a way that suits you best. I want you to get the most you can from this program and have the best life you desire and deserve. I invite you use your resources to apply the practices to your daily life so you will always be prepared for life's storms. What you need to do next is get clear and committed to how you will keep doing this program to take advantage of your anxiety and be empowered. You can do it on your own if you have the perseverance and the resources and a great plan. It is my experience that people who continue supporting themselves with coaching are more successful at reaching their goals. The women I have walked with through my 9-week Fear-Less program and my 13-month Make It Your Own ongoing coaching program have the experience, knowledge, and practices in their bones and are making absolutely amazing changes in their lives. Anxiety is their advantage now as a warning sign for them to pay attention to what is happening inside. It never gets to take over again in the same old way.

I have come through my own anxiety challenges, and it never stops me now from taking the risks I choose to take. Writing this book and putting this program online is another huge leap for me. It has been a truly life-changing gift. I feel compelled to share this program with a bigger audience and help as many people as I can.

I am so grateful every day for staying on my path and securing my daily practice so that I can keep creating the next dream to live. Life is amazing and precious. I intend to stay conscious of that. Now it is your turn. I know you can do it. You know it is possible to live without anxiety running you after reading this book. Now it is time to digest it, practice it, and live it.

I invite you to stay in touch. As part of being a reader of my book, I want you to keep in touch with me through my website www.katedow.com.

I truly want you to get the most you can from this program and have the life you have been waiting for.

Always be True to Yourself,

Dr. Kate Dow

REFERENCES

Introduction

1. www.calm.clinic.com with NIMH statistics on anxiety disorders prevalence.

2. Shields, GS; Kuchenbecker, SY; Pressman, SD; Sumida, KD; Slavich, GM. "Better cognitive control of emotional information is associated with reduced pro-inflammatory cytokine reactivity to emotional stress," Stress. (2016, 19(1):63-8.)

3. Jung, CG. *The Concept of the Collective Unconscious* (CW. Vol 9, part 1, pp. 42-53.)

4. Bolen, Jean Shiboda. *Goddesses in Everywoman: Powerful Archetypes in Women's Lives* (New York: Harper, 1984), p. 29.

5. Hadjibalassi, M; Lambrinou, E; Papastavrou, E; Papathanassoglou, E. "The effect of guided imagery on physiological and psychological outcomes of adult ICU patients: A systematic literature review and methodological implications." Aust Crit Care.

(2017 Mar 29.) (pii: S1036-7314(17)30164-9. doi: 10.1016/j.aucc.2017.03.001.)

6. Jacquart, J; Miller, KM; Radossi, A; Haime, V; Macklin, E; Gilburd, D; Nelson Oliver, M; Mehta, DH; Yeung, A; Fricchione, GL; Benson, H; Denninger, JW. "The effectiveness of a community-based, mind-body group for symptoms of depression and anxiety." Adv Mind Body Med. (2014 Summer; 28(3):6-13)

7. Como, JM. "Spiritual practice: A literature review related to spiritual health and health outcomes." Holist Nurs Pract (2007 Sep-Oct; 21(5):224-36.)

Chapter Two

1. Swiftdeer, Reagan, Harley *Sweet Medicine Sundance Teachings of the Chuluaqui-Quodoushka* (California, The Deer Tribe Metis-Medicine Society 1986.)

2. Ruiz, Don Miguel *The Four Agreements* (San Rafael, Aber-Allen Publishing, Inc.,1997)

3. www.postpartum.net – Postpartum Support International

4. www.alanon.com – The Alanon Program

5. www.purestpotential.com – Santa Fe Yoga

6. www.tantraheart.com – Tantra Heart

7. www.awakeningwoman.com – Chameli Ardagh

8. www.pemachodron.com – Pema Chodron

9. www.dharmaocean – Reggie Ray

Chapter Four

1. Bolen, Jean Shiboda Goddesses in Everywoman: Powerful Archetypes in Women's Lives. (New York: Harper,1984)
2. Williamson, Marianne. A Women's Worth (Toronto: Random House, 1993)

Chapter Five

1. Avinasha, Bodhi *The Ipsalu Formula: A Method for Tantra Bliss* (United States: Ipsalu Publishing, 2003)
2. Wilkes C, Kydd R, Sagar M, Broadbent E. Upright posture improves affect and fatigue in people with depressive symptoms.(J Behav Ther Exp Psychiatry. 2017 Mar;54:143-149. doi: 10.1016/j.jbtep.2016.07.015. Epub 2016 Jul 30.)

Chapter Six

1. Brown AJ, Sun CC, Urbauer DL, Bodurka DC, Thaker PH, Ramondetta LM. Feeling powerless: Locus of control as a potential target for supportive care interventions to increase quality of life and decrease anxiety in ovarian cancer patients. (Gynecol Oncol. 2015 Aug;138(2):388-93.) doi: 10.1016/j.ygyno.2015.05.005. Epub 2015 May 16.)
2. Carter LW, Mollen D, Smith NG.Locus of control, minority stress, and psychological distress among lesbian, gay, and bisexual individuals. (J Couns Psychol. 2014 Jan;61(1):169-75. doi: 10.1037/a0034593. Epub 2013 Nov 4.)

3. Panno A, Carrus G, Lafortezza R, Mariani L, Sanesi G. Nature-based solutions to promote human resilience and wellbeing in cities during increasingly hot summers. (Environ Res. 2017 Aug 16;159:249-256. doi: 10.1016/j.envres.2017.08.016.)

4. Oschman JL, Chevalier G, Brown R. The effects of grounding (earthing) on inflammation, the immune response, wound healing, and prevention and treatment of chronic inflammatory and autoimmune diseases.(J Inflamm Res. 2015 Mar 24;8:83-96. doi: 10.2147/JIR. S69656. eCollection 2015.)

5. Fujitani T, Ohara K, Kouda K, Mase T, Miyawaki C, Momoi K, Okita Y, Furutani M, Nakamura H. Association of social support with gratitude and sense of coherence in Japanese young women: a cross-sectional study. (Psychol Res Behav Manag. 2017 Jun 27;10:195-200. doi: 10.2147/PRBM. S137374. eCollection 2017.)

6. Pérez-Farinós N, Villar-Villalba C, López Sobaler AM, Dal Re Saavedra MÁ, Aparicio A, Santos Sanz S, Robledo de Dios T, Castrodeza-Sanz JJ, Ortega Anta RM. The relationship between hours of sleep, screen time and frequency of food and drink consumption in Spain in the 2011 and 2013 ALADINO: a cross-sectional study. (BMC Public Health. 2017 Jan 6;17(1):33. doi: 10.1186/s12889-016-3962-4.)

Chapter Seven

1. Ruiz, Don Miguel. *The Four Agreements* (San Rafael, Aber-Allen Publishing, Inc., 1997).

Chapter Eight

1. Marija, Gimbutas. "Women and Culture in Goddess-Oriented Old Europe," in *The politics of Women's Spirituality; Essays on the Rise of Spiritual Power within the Women's Movement*, ed. Charlene Spretnak (New York: Doubleday, 1982 (pp. 22-31).

2. Petevari J, Osman M, Bhattacharya J. The Role of Intuition in the Generation and Evaluation Stages of Creativity. (Front Psychol 2016 Sep 20;7:1420. eCollection 2016.)

3. Wolever, RQ; Bobinet, KJ; McCabe, K; Mackenzie, ER; Feket, e E; Kusnick, CA; Baime, M. Effective and viable mind-body stress reduction in the workplace: a randomized controlled trial. (J Occup Health Psychol. 2012 Apr;17(2):246-58. doi: 10.1037/a0027278. Epub 2012 Feb 20.)

Chapter Nine

1. Dugan AG, Barnes-Farrell JL. Time for Self-Care: Downtime Recovery as a Buffer of Work and Home/Family Time Pressures. (J Occup Environ Med. 2017 Apr;59(4):e46-e56. doi: 10.1097/JOM.0000000000000975.)

2. Hay ME, Connelly DM, Kinsella EA. Embodiment and aging in contemporary physiotherapy

(Physiother Theory Pract.32(4):241-50) doi: 10.3109/09593985.2016.1138348.)

3. Kontos P, Martin W. Embodiment and dementia: exploring critical narratives of selfhood, surveillance, and dementia care. (Dementia (London). 2013 May;12(3):288-302. doi: 10.1177/1471301213479787. Epub 2013 Mar 7.)

4. Chevalier G. The effect of grounding the human body on mood. (Psychol Rep. 2015 Apr;116(2):534-42. doi: 10.2466/06.PR0.116k21w5. Epub 2015 Mar 6.)

5. Oschman JL, Chevalier G, Brown R. The effects of grounding (earthing) on inflammation, the immune response, wound healing, and prevention and treatment of chronic inflammatory and autoimmune diseases. (J Inflamm Res, 2015 Mar 24;8:83-96. doi: 10.2147/JIR. S69656. eCollection 2015.)

6. Bhajan, Yogi The Aquarian Teacher (Kundalini Research Institute, 2003)

7. Doll A, Hölzel BK, Mulej Bratec S, Boucard CC, Xie X, Wohlschläger AM, Sorg C Mindful attention to breath regulates emotions via increased amygdala-prefrontal cortex connectivity. (Neuroimage 2016 Jul 1;134:305-313. doi: 10.1016/j.neuroimage.2016.03.041) Epub 2016 Mar 24.)

8. Cho H, Ryu S, Noh J, Lee J. The Effectiveness of Daily Mindful Breathing Practices on Test Anxiety of Students. (Plos One 2016 Oct 20;11(10):e0164822. doi:.1371/journal.pone.0164822. eCollection 2016.)

9.   Brown RP, Gerbarg PL. Sudarshan Kriya yogic breathing in the treatment of stress, anxiety, and depression: part I-neurophysiologic model. (J Altern Complement Med. 2005 Feb;11(1):189-201.)

Chapter Ten

1.   Arora S, Ashrafian H, Davis R, Athanasiou T, Darzi A, Sevdalis N. Emotional intelligence in medicine: a systematic review through the context of the ACGME competencies. (Med 2010 Aug;44(8):749-64. doi: 10.1111/j.1365-2923.2010.03709.x.)

2.   Schutte N., Malouf J. et al. Emotional Intelligence and Interpersonal Relations. (J of Soc Psych, 2001 Vol 141, Iss 4, pgs 523-536.)

3.   Palmer B, Donaldson C., Stough C Emotional Intelligence and Life Satisfaction. (Pers and Ind Diff 2002, Vol 33 Iss 7 pg 1091-1100.)

4.   Sarno, John MD The Mind-Body Prescription: Healing the Body, Healing the Pain. (US, Time Warner Company, 1998)

5.   Esteves JE, Wheatley L, Mayall C, Abbey H. Emotional processing and its relationship to chronic low back pain: results from a case-control study. (Man Ther. 2013 Dec;18(6):541-6. doi: 10.1016/j.math.2013.05.008. Epub 2013 Jun)

6.   Perlman SD. Psychoanalytic treatment of chronic pain: the body speaks on multiple levels. (J Am Psychoanal 1996 Summer;24(2):257-71.)

Chapter Eleven

1. Dundas I, Binder PE, Hansen TGB, Stige SH. Does a short self-compassion intervention for students increase healthy self-regulation? A randomized control trial. (Scand J Psychol 2017 Aug 28. doi: 10.1111/sjop.12385. [Epub ahead of print])

2. Orellana-Rios CL, Radbruch L, Kern M, Regel YU, Anton A, Sinclair S, Schmidt S. Mindfulness and compassion-oriented practices at work reduce distress and enhance self-care of palliative care teams: a mixed-method evaluation of an "on the job" program. (BMC Palliat Care. 2017 Jul 6;17(1):3. doi: 10.1186/s12904-017-0219-7.)

3. www.hooponopono.org

4. https://pennebaker.socialpsychology.org/

Chapter Thirteen

1. Fujitani T, Ohara K, Kouda K, Mase T, Miyawaki C, Momoi K, Okita Y, Furutani M, Nakamura H. Association of social support with gratitude and sense of coherence in Japanese young women: a cross-sectional study. (Psychol Res Behav Manag. 2017 Jun 27;10:195-200. doi: 10.2147/PRBM. S137374. eCollection 2017.)

2. Kyeong S, Kim J, Kim DJ, Kim HE, Kim JJ. Effects of gratitude meditation on neural network functional connectivity and brain-heart coupling. (Sci Rep. 2017 Jul 11;7(1):5058. doi: 10.1038/s41598-017-05520-9.)

3. Mill P, Redwine L, Wilson K et.al. The Role of Gratitude in Spiritual Well-being in Asymptomatic Heart Failure Patients. (Spiritual Clin Pract. 2015 Mar; 2(1): 5–7. doi: 10.1037/scp0000050.)

4. Chodron, Pema *The Places that Scare you: A Guide to Fearlessness in Difficult Times.* (Boston, Shambhala, 2002)

5. Bhajan Yogi *The Aquarian Teacher* (Kundalini Research Institute 2003)

6. Telles S, Gupta RK, Yadav A, Pathak S, Balkrishna A. Hemisphere specific EEG related to alternate nostril yoga breathing. (BMC Res Notes. 2017 Jul 24;10(1):306. doi: 10.1186/s13104-017-2625-6.)

Chapter Fourteen

1. www.tarabrach.com

2. Görg N, Priebe K, Böhnke JR, Steil R, Dyer AS, Kleindienst N. Trauma-related emotions and radical acceptance in dialectical behavior therapy for posttraumatic stress disorder after childhood sexual abuse. (Borderline Personal Disord Emot Dysregul. 2017 Jul 13;4:15. doi: 10.1186/s40479-017-0065-5. eCollection 2017.)

3. Kearney DJ, Malte CA, McManus C, Martinez ME, Felleman B, Simpson TL. Loving-kindness meditation for posttraumatic stress disorder: a pilot study. (J Trauma Stress. 2013 Aug;26(4):426-34. doi: 10.1002/jts.21832. Epub 2013 Jul 25.)

4. Feliu-Soler A, Pascual JC, Elices M, Martín-Blanco A, Carmona C, Cebolla A, Simón V, Soler J. Fostering Self-Compassion and Loving-Kindness in Patients With Borderline Personality Disorder: A Randomized Pilot Study. (Clin Psychol Psychother. 2017 Jan;24(1):278-286. doi: 10.1002/cpp.2000. Epub 2016 Jan 28.)

5. Chodron, Pema *The Places that Scare you: A Guide to Fearlessness in Difficult Times.* (Boston, Shambhala, 2002)

Chapter Fifteen

1. Koslander T, da Silva AB, Roxberg A. Existential and spiritual needs in mental health care: an ethical and holistic perspective. (J Holist Nurs. 2009 Mar;27(1):34-42. doi: 10.1177/0898010108323302. Epub 2009 Jan 28.)

2. Seaward BL. Stress and human spirituality 2000: at the cross roads of physics and metaphysics. (Appl Psychophysiol Biofeedback. 2000 Dec;25(4):241-6.)

3. Lin HR Bauer-Wu SM. Psycho-spiritual well-being in patients with advanced cancer: an integrative review of the literature.(J Adv Nurs. 2003 Oct;44(1):69-80.)

4. Cahn BR, Goodman MS, Peterson CT, Maturi R, Mills PJ. Yoga, Meditation and Mind-Body Health: Increased BDNF, Cortisol Awakening Response, and Altered Inflammatory Marker Expression after a 3-Month Yoga and Meditation Retreat. (Front Hum Neurosci. 2017 Jun 26;11:315. doi: 10.3389/fnhum.2017.00315. eCollection 2017.)

5. Campanella F, Crescentini C, Urgesi C, Fabbro F. Mindfulness-oriented meditation improves self-related character scales in healthy individuals. (Compr Psychiatry. 2014 Jul;55(5):1269-78. doi: 10.1016/j. comppsych.2014.03.009. Epub 2014 Mar 26.)

ACKNOWLEDGMENTS

First, I want to acknowledge the totality of people, circumstances, and experiences of my life as my ultimate teachers, bringing me to where I am now. I accept, honor, and appreciate them all.

I am grateful to each and every one of my clients who have allowed me to support them on their journeys, which infinitely served my skills, experience and growth. A special thank you to my program clients for sharing in the creation of this book: Juana, Erin, Gabrielle, Sharon, and Tracy.

I want to acknowledge my wonderful teachers who have profoundly helped me to evolve and awaken into myself: Dr. Liz Chandra of Sweet Medicine Sundance Path, Don Miguel Ruiz of the Toltec Tradition, Kirn and GC Khalsa of Santa Fe Yoga Kundalini, Chameli Ardagh of Awakening Women, Pema Chodron, Reggie Ray of Dharma Ocean, and Richard and Antoinette Assimus of Tantra Heart. My deep gratitude and love to my inner spiritual teachers and Divine Mother, Mother Earth, Father Sky, and Creator of All That Is.

To the Morgan James Publishing team: Special thanks to David Hancock, CEO & Founder for believing in me and my message. To my Author Relations Manager, Tiffany Gibson, thanks for making the process seamless and easy. Many more thanks to everyone else, but especially Jim Howard, Bethany Marshall, and Nickcole Watkins.

Thank you to my mother and father for all of your love and support. I thank my dear friends who have been with me through the many phases of my life, caring, loving and being there for me. I want to especially acknowledge my son Gabriel and my daughter Amara, who have been my greatest teachers, my dear family, and my greatest inspiration to keep growing. Thank you for helping me become my best version of myself and putting up with me at my worst. And I thank my own Soul for lovingly nudging me along in the face of adversity and human suffering to unveil my True Self.

ABOUT THE AUTHOR

Dr. Kate Dow is an author, facilitator, speaker and mentor. For over 30 years, she has been passionate about her work with women as a psychologist and life coach. She has been a lifetime seeker of what truly helps people to heal, recover and generate a life of personal growth, empowerment 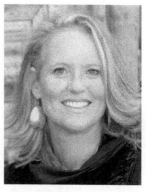 and wholeness. She is always learning and opening to what life offers to be of service to others in the best way possible.

Dr. Kate has extensively studied mind-body medicine for three decades. She has a PhD in Counseling Psychology and is a Certified Wellness Coach and Kundalini Yoga Teacher. She closely apprenticed in Toltec Traditions for eight years with Don Miguel Ruiz, the author of *The Four Agreements*. She is a Level 5 Kriya Yoga practitioner of Tantric Arts and Reiki level two practitioner. She has studied Tibetan Buddhism for the past

10 years, and currently trains with Dharma Ocean in Somatic Meditation.

What Dr. Kate loves the most is bringing together the wisdom of traditional teachings with current mind-body scientific research and newer healing modalities to create unique, well-informed, and powerful online programs and in-person retreats that are transformational and life-changing for women.

Dr. Kate, the CEO of Sacred Transitions, Inc., formed her center in 1995 to provide a place for powerful change for women in practical, compassionate ways. She is an adoring mother of her two amazing teenagers, Gabriel and Amara; her two dogs, Daphne and Bodhi; and her black cat, Jack. She continues to feel blessed to live in Santa Fe, New Mexico.

Website: www.katedow.com

Email: katedowphd@gmail.com

Phone: 505-577-8042

THANK YOU

I appreciate you for being here.

Let's keep Stepping into Empowerment!

Thank you so much for reading *Fear-Less: The Art of Using Anxiety to Your Advantage*. I would love to hear about your experience, if you want to email me at katedowphd@gmail.com.

I am so excited to share this passion for a fear-less life with you. It is so vital that we know life can be different, especially for female entrepreneurs who want to get their message out there. Getting this book gives you the initial exposure to these teachings and tools. What I have found is that, unless you have the right support to keep putting these practices into action, most people will not receive the full bounty of awe-inspiring benefits that are available to them in this program.

To help make this happen, I am offering many way to keep growing, learing and evolving on my website www.katedow.com.

If you have enjoyed this book, please write a review on Amazon and post a picture of you with the book on Facebook or Instagram. I really want to hear from you! Keep taking advantage of your anxiety and using it to become powerful YOU again!

(A portion of the profit of this book will be donated to programs that support women in health, education, and financial independence.)

With Great Courage and Compassion,

Dr. Kate Dow

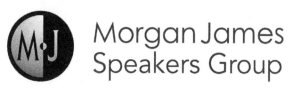

Morgan James
Speakers Group

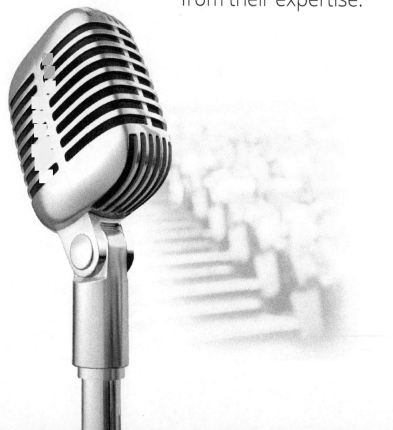

↗ www.TheMorganJamesSpeakersGroup.com

We connect Morgan James published
authors with live and online events
and audiences who will benefit
from their expertise.

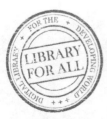

Printed in the USA
CPSIA information can be obtained
at www.ICGtesting.com
JSHW022340140824
68134JS00019B/1590